Praise for *The Emotional Eater's Repair Manual*

"A must-read for anyone who struggles with overeating. Julie Simon offers a beautifully written, compassion-filled guide for ending emotional eating, yo-yo dieting, and poor health. She'll show you how to nurture yourself with loving behaviors and wholesome foods and address your soul's yearnings for joy and fulfillment. Her message is both practical and inspirational."

— Rory Freedman, coauthor of *Skinny Bitch*

"If you are like most of us, you eat for many different reasons — to fuel your body, of course, but also for comfort, excitement, distraction, and companionship and to satisfy other emotional needs. In this marvelous book, Julie Simon takes you on a journey of self-care and soul-care that will help you understand your emotional and spiritual hungers, heal your relationship with food, and bring balance and happiness into your life."

— John Robbins, author of *The Food Revolution*,
Diet for a New America, and *No Happy Cows*

"Nearly every woman I know (including myself) has collapsed into cycles of emotional eating, and then later felt ashamed about it. Our compulsive striving for perfection, acceptance, and love from others can cause us to feel continually 'not good enough,' depleted, and empty. In the black hole of our loneliness and pain we then turn to food to fill and soothe us. Thank goodness that Julie M. Simon's *The Emotional Eater's Repair Manual* teaches women another way. This is a compassionate and intelligent guide that can help women step out of this vicious cycle by listening to their intuition instead of counting calories. By addressing all aspects of a woman's inner and outer life — from her brain chemistry to the robustness of her social and spiritual connectedness — Simon's anti-diet approach gives women the tools they need to *finally* feel comfortable in their own skin."

— Sara Avant Stover, author of *The Way of the Happy Woman*

"So many people struggle with emotional eating and the problems it causes. In *The Emotional Eater's Repair Manual*, you will find the step-by-step solution you've been looking for. Reassuring and calm, informative and inspiring, this book is your lifeline to fixing your relationship with food and gaining the health you deserve."

— Neal D. Barnard, MD, president,
Physicians Committee for Responsible Medicine, Washington, DC,
and author of *Breaking the Food Seduction* and
Dr. Neal Barnard's Program for Reversing Diabetes

"An invaluable book that addresses the true underlying causes of overeating and weight gain. *The Emotional Eater's Repair Manual* breaks new ground and offers a fresh, heartfelt approach to an age-old problem. Highly recommended!"

— Hyla Cass, MD, author of *8 Weeks to Vibrant Health*

"[Julie Simon] writes with the compassion of a survivor as she shares the Twelve-Week Emotional Eating Recovery Program she created.... Simon doesn't make quick-fix promises but she does assure readers that, at their own pace and according to their own terms, they can free themselves from emotional overeating, and that weight loss will follow naturally.... This book is truly unique. It packages a complete system for inner and outer change in nurturing, realistic terms with specific directions that move readers toward their goals."

— Anna Jedrziewski, *Retailing Insight*

THE EMOTIONAL EATER'S REPAIR MANUAL

THE EMOTIONAL EATER'S REPAIR MANUAL

A Practical Mind-Body-Spirit Guide
for Putting an End to Overeating and Dieting

JULIE M. SIMON

MA, MBA, LMFT

New World Library
Novato, California

New World Library
14 Pamaron Way
Novato, California 94949

Text design by Tona Pearce Myers

Library of Congress Cataloging-in-Publication Data
Simon, Julie M., 1956–
    The emotional eater's repair manual : a practical mind-body-spirit guide for putting an end to overeating and dieting / Julie M. Simon, MA, MBA.
        p.   cm.
Includes bibliographical references and index.
ISBN 978-1-60868-151-8 (pbk. : alk. paper)
    1. Eating disorders—Psychological aspects. 2. Diet—Psychological aspects. 3. Nutrition. I. Title.
RC552.E18S56 2012
616.85'26—dc23   2012030685

First printing, November 2012
ISBN 978-1-60868-151-8
Printed in Canada on 100% postconsumer-waste recycled paper

New World Library is proud to be a Gold Certified Environmentally Responsible Publisher. Publisher certification awarded by Green Press Initiative. www.greenpressinitiative.org

10   9   8   7   6   5   4   3   2

To Mamakitty, my soul mate and the best writing companion ever.
Rest in peace, sweetheart.

CONTENTS

Introduction

If you've picked up this book, most likely you're regularly overeating comfort foods and battling your weight. You're probably sick and tired of dealing with this issue, and you may literally be *sick and tired* from your overeating. Perhaps you already have some health conditions that you fear might be related to your eating and weight. Does it feel as if stress and a hectic lifestyle derail your best intentions — leading you to grab unhealthy processed foods loaded with sugar and fat and overeat at meals? Are you drinking beverages like soda and coffee to keep going? Join the club.

You've probably tried many eating and exercise plans but have always found it difficult to stick with them. Or maybe you've had some success with a particular program and are wondering why you always slip back to eating your favorite foods and gaining back the weight. Perhaps you've come to believe that you lack willpower or discipline, and this makes you feel ashamed and guilty. Take heart; you're not alone.

I know firsthand how frustrating overeating and gaining weight can be. I spent a good portion of my life stuck in a cycle of overeating comfort foods, gaining weight, and dieting. My health was suffering. I was never good at sticking with diet plans — in fact, I always felt food-obsessed the minute I put myself on a diet. Whenever I did muster the motivation to go on another diet, I would lose a small amount of weight and then plateau. While each new diet plan restored some hope and motivation, compulsive food cravings and a sense of restriction and deprivation always led me back to overeating and weight gain.

I know that I definitely ate emotionally — I used food to calm and soothe myself. It helped numb the pain of unpleasant emotions, self-doubts and other negative thoughts, and general stress. Food altered my brain chemistry; and because food is pleasurable and exciting, it was a good distraction. It temporarily filled up the inner emptiness and restlessness I regularly felt, a sort of spiritual hunger.

I found it especially difficult to stay away from comfort foods like bread, muffins, chips, cookies, scones, ice cream, and candy, and beverages like diet soda and coffee. You would think that once I was losing weight and feeling better while *off* these substances, I would *stay* off of them. *You would think*. I knew my body didn't *need* them; but I *wanted* them. Does this sound familiar?

Throughout my years of emotional eating and weight challenges, I was afraid my body was telling me that I was one of those unfortunate people who would have to live the rest of her life on a low-calorie diet or remain overweight. I was concerned that chronic dieting would harm my metabolism, and I was worried that the "or remain overweight" would be my future. I knew I wasn't one of those people who could eat *anything* and stay slim, but I also knew that maintaining my weight shouldn't be so hard.

My mind, body, and spirit were trying to tell me something. It took many years of study, therapy, and visits to health care practitioners for me to understand and resolve all the pieces of the overeating puzzle in my own life. As each piece of the puzzle fell into place, my life got better and better. I no longer felt compulsive about food. My weight and mood stabilized. I felt less overwhelmed. I procrastinated less. My inner chaos and outer clutter diminished. I felt more emotionally balanced than I had ever been in my life. A nourishing inner voice was developing, and with it, self-acceptance and self-love. Connection and intimacy were replacing the emptiness and loneliness I had lived with for so long.

Looking back, I can see that my emotional eating and weight problems were actually a blessing in disguise, symptoms bothersome enough to push me to look for an internal solution rather than another diet. In the process, I *lost* all the excess weight and, more important, I *gained* the skills needed to take the best care of myself *for life*. And you can too. No more emotional eating. No more overeating. No more weight gain. No more dieting. There is a better way.

Mind-Body-Spirit Balance

You were born with a phenomenal mind, body, and spirit that give you a multitude of signals everyday. Emotional signals, like feelings of joy, happiness, love, and contentment, and cognitive signals, like empowering, positive, pleasant thoughts, let you know that your inner world is calm and serene. Physical signals like hunger, thirst, cravings, and fullness guide you to take the best care of your body and stay in balance. And spiritual signals like inspiration, purpose, and passion inform you that you're taking good care of your soul.

Signals that are out of the ordinary, such as compulsive food cravings, weight gain, fatigue, inflammation, and pain, are your body's way of telling you something's out of balance. Chronic anxiety, depression, or hopelessness, and persistent negative, critical, fear-based thoughts, are your mind's way of alerting you to imbalance. Loneliness, emptiness, purposelessness, boredom, and apathy are your spirit's way of giving you a wake-up call.

Most likely you've lost some of this intuitive connection to yourself and you're feeling imbalanced. Perhaps you've lost touch with your signals on many levels, and when symptoms surface you ignore or medicate them. You find yourself unable to practice suggested lifestyle changes or address health challenges because of an emotional, physical, and spiritual disconnect that sabotages your best intentions.

Proper nutrition and regular exercise are important aspects of losing and maintaining weight, but they're only part of the weight loss equation.

Most diet books and weight loss programs focus exclusively on reduced-calorie eating plans and exercise regimens. They attempt to apply external solutions to internal problems.

We all love to eat, and enjoying food beyond simple sustenance is a normal part of life. It becomes problematic when we overeat to such an extent that there is a significant weight gain or health risk. Overeating may seem like a simple act, but it's actually a complex behavior. Its resolution requires a comprehensive, multidimensional approach.

When we eat in the absence of physical hunger cues, regularly choose unhealthy comfort foods, or eat when we're already full, something is out of balance somewhere.

These tendencies may represent imbalance in any of the following three areas: the mind, the body, and the spirit.

The Mind

Imbalances in this area can result from any of the following:

- Chronic unpleasant emotions
- Unmet needs
- Lack of an internalized nurturing voice
- Negative, critical, fearful, self-defeating thoughts
- Unresolved pain from childhood
- Ineffective limit and boundary setting
- Lack of self-acceptance and self-love

And these can lead to overeating driven by an exaggerated desire for pleasure, soothing, comfort, fulfillment, excitement, and distraction.

The Body

Imbalances in this area may be due to any of the following:

- Chronic dieting
- Overconsumption of processed foods and foods of animal origin
- Hormonal irregularities
- Low or high brain chemicals
- Food allergies and sensitivities

- Environmental toxins
- Stress and a fast-paced, sedentary lifestyle

And these can lead to food cravings, low energy, and poor sleep, creating a vicious cycle of comfort eating, weight gain, and more dieting.

The Spirit

Imbalances in this area may result from any of the following:

- Busyness or a restless mind
- Control issues
- Lack of purpose or meaning
- Loneliness

And these can lead to overeating as an attempt to fill up spiritual reserves.

You *Can* End Your Emotional Eating without Going on Another Diet

If you're ready for an alternative to dieting, this book is for you. It will help you address the true causes of your overeating or imbalanced eating. I won't ask you to count calories or weigh and measure food. Nor will I suggest exhausting workout routines. Your body has a natural weight, not overweight and not underweight. Maintaining this weight should be easy, comfortable, and intuitive.

Your mind, body, and spirit may be screaming that they're out of balance. This book is your repair manual. It's your guide to learning and practicing self- and soul-care skills and body-balancing principles that will help you reconnect to yourself, pay attention to your signals, and respond appropriately to meet your needs without turning to food for comfort, soothing, distraction, excitement, and so on.

A Unique Approach

This may not be the first book you've turned to for help with your over-eating. So what makes this approach unique?

This approach is comprehensive: it covers the emotional, physical, and spiritual imbalances that underlie overeating. In my twenty-plus years of practice, I've observed firsthand the intricate relationship between mind, body, and spirit. For example, I see that stressful urban lifestyles lead us to grab unhealthy processed foods and beverages that take a toll on our bodies and, in turn, deplete our emotional and spiritual reserves. Similarly, I've noticed that overeaters raised in dysfunctional family environments have an emotionally and spiritually starved inner child running the show. They often lack the most basic skills that would allow them to naturally and effortlessly care for their bodies.

In part 1 of this book, you'll learn

- the emotional and cognitive/behavioral mind signals that inform you whether your inner world is in or out of balance; and
- the five basic self-care skills you may not have acquired in childhood, or later in adult life, that enable you to pay attention to your signals, take the best care of yourself, and maintain balance; deficits in any of these skills can result in emotional eating.

In part 2, you'll learn

- the body signals that guide you in deciding when to eat, what to eat, how much to eat, and when to stop eating;
- the most natural and nutritious eating plan consistent with your human design, one that does not create further imbalance;
- the body and brain signals highlighting a biochemical imbalance that can lead to low energy, food cravings, and overeating;
- the importance of moving your body and getting enough sleep; and
- the five principles of balanced biochemistry that will keep your body functioning optimally.

In part 3, you'll learn

- the psychospiritual signals such as restlessness, purposelessness, and loneliness that can lead to emotional eating; and
- the five soul-care practices that will assist you in keeping your spiritual reserves full.

The truth is, you *can* put an end to emotional eating and dieting forever. I did, and I will show you how. While there is no quick fix to resolving years of overeating, the skills, principles, and practices outlined in this book, when followed, will bring about changes right away that will motivate and encourage you to continue.

This approach can be customized to meet your individual needs. Emotional eaters come in many different sizes, shapes, and backgrounds. Any successful weight loss program must have enough structure to yield reliable, consistent results *and* be flexible enough that you can adapt it to your individual needs.

The skills, principles, and practices detailed in each part of the book apply across the board to everyone. Some you may already be practicing. Others you may not need to implement if, in that particular area, you exhibit no symptoms of imbalance. And others are the key skills, principles, or practices that, when mastered, will resolve your unique emotional-eating challenge.

While this program works best when you correct all or most of your particular areas of imbalance, mastering even one skill, or practicing just one principle, and incorporating the changes into your lifestyle can provide some relief from emotional eating.

The skills, principles, and practices outlined in this program can be utilized for life to quickly restore balance. Life is a constant balancing act. Just when we feel in balance, something occurs to throw us back out of balance. Travel, stress, illness, financial challenges, losses, and disappointments all have their way of derailing our best intentions. This repair manual will be your lifelong resource for identifying and resolving areas of imbalance. You can focus on select skills, principles, or practices whenever you fall off the wagon.

How to Use This Book

This is a self-help book adapted from my Twelve-Week Emotional Eating Recovery Program. Although it's designed to let you proceed from part 1 to part 2 to part 3, feel free to skip around and read first the parts that interest you the most.

We begin addressing emotional eating by building the skills needed to take the best care of ourselves. It's best to practice the skills in part 1 in the order given, if possible, because the associated exercises build on the exercises that precede them. While you will benefit from simply reading about the skills, the exercises will increase self-awareness and help you build these skills, shift your attitudes, and heal old wounds. Some of the exercises may arouse strong, uncomfortable emotions. You may want to work through them with a friend (or friends) who is challenged by the same or similar issues. Doing so can provide support, comfort, and encouragement as you continue through the program.

If you find you're encountering internal resistance and lack the motivation to practice all the exercises provided in part 1, do the ones you can for now. You can always go back and do more of them at a later date. Lack of motivation or willingness may highlight blocked emotional areas. Slowly working through these areas of imbalance will most likely unlock the key to your resistance. Remember to be gentle with yourself; there are many roads leading to recovery.

In part 2, we focus on clearing out any biochemical imbalances that lead to unhealthy eating habits. If you can reduce or eliminate compulsive food cravings, bingeing, bloating, unpleasant mood fluctuations, fatigue, and low energy caused by physical imbalances, you'll get a clearer picture of how much of your overeating is driven by emotional and spiritual hunger. If you find you can easily address the physical imbalances, and this resolves your eating issues, then you may be one of the lucky few who simply need a biochemical tune-up.

It may feel easier and more motivating to start in part 2, addressing your body and brain imbalances first, and then go back and address the skill building in part 1. If you feel stalled on any principle, you can always begin practicing the next one and then go back later to an earlier one. If you're already practicing a particular principle — for example, you already have an exercise plan that you're satisfied with — feel free to skip my discussion of that principle. Some of the principles you can practice immediately, some will require more time, and others may require you to work with a health care provider.

In part 3, we complete our work by addressing the psychospiritual imbalances underlying overeating. In this section, feel free to skip around and read the practices that are of particular interest to you.

It will take time to build the skills, practice the principles, and apply the practices outlined in this book and to integrate them into your life. Allow yourself the time you need to proceed through the three parts of this book. You can go as fast or as slowly as you like. *There truly is no rush.* You did not become an emotional eater overnight, and your eating issues will not go away overnight. Watch any tendency toward perfectionism, which may imbalance you further. It's more important to consistently — not perfectly — practice what you're learning. A slow and steady approach is generally the most prudent way to conquer your emotional eating and meet your weight loss goals.

Whether you want to lose a large amount of weight, end a compulsive overeating problem, stop obsessing about food and weight, shed those last few pounds, or just improve your health, this program offers you exactly what you need: information, examples, clinically proven techniques, guidance, and encouragement. There's no time like the present to get started.

PART ONE

Mastering Self-Care Skills

CHAPTER ONE

When Overeating Is Driven by Emotional Hunger

People come to my seminars, workshops, groups, and Twelve-Week Emotional Eating Recovery Program because they feel they've done everything they can to stop overeating and lose weight. They've tried diets, fasts, exercise regimens, pills, shots, hypnosis, gastric bypass, lap-band surgery, and alternative health care practices, all to no avail. They've lost weight and gained it back, and they still can't stop overeating. Referred by their friends, family members, colleagues, physicians, dietitians, and other health care providers, they come to see me in a confused and desperate state — they feel like I am their last hope. Some are obese; some are suffering from multiple degenerative conditions such as diabetes and high blood pressure. Others are closer to their goal weight but can't stop thinking about food and fatness. They believe they lack willpower. They label themselves as lazy, undisciplined, or powerless, primarily when it comes to eating and exercise.

Many emotional eaters believe that their weight challenges are the result of factors outside their control.

> "Everyone in my family is heavy; it's just my genetics and there's nothing I can do besides severe dieting."
> "There's no time to exercise while working full-time and raising a family."

"There's constantly food around at my job, and most of it is high
in fat and junky; it's just too tempting."

"Socially, we eat out regularly in restaurants, and it's nearly impossible to eat healthfully without offending others."

"Ever since I injured my foot, I've packed on the pounds. I can't
do heavy-duty cardio like I used to."

"I overeat just because I love food and eating."

While these factors are reasonable and do play a part in our overeating, they *do not* represent the true cause of our inability to take weight
off and keep it off. We all have a natural body weight, and our bodies are
not naturally overweight or underweight. Maintaining this weight is supposed to be easy, comfortable, and intuitive.

We all enjoy eating and, on occasion, will eat when not hungry or
overeat just because the food is incredibly tasty or because it enhances our
personal or social experiences. An afternoon out with a good friend is certainly more enjoyable with coffee and a pastry. And what would a good
movie be without a bag of popcorn? There's nothing wrong with occasionally using food to enhance enjoyment and celebrate life. The problem
arises when we use food in this way so often that we become overweight
or our health is at risk.

The truth is, if you regularly eat when you're not hungry or when
you're already full, or if you regularly choose to eat unhealthy comfort
foods, the bulk of your overeating occurs *not* just because you love food
and enjoy eating or have a stressful schedule. And it's not because you're
lazy and undisciplined, have bad genes, or lack willpower. Your emotional eating represents your limited ability to care for yourself. It's a sign
that you're lacking self-care skills that are generally learned in childhood.
Emotional eating highlights your difficulty in connecting to yourself;
in paying attention to your mind, body, and spirit signals; and in responding appropriately to meet your needs. As disturbing as this may sound, it
is true.

What do I mean when I say *mind*, *body*, and *spirit signals*? I'm talking about emotional signals, such as joy, happiness, sadness, and anger. And cognitive signals, like pleasant, empowering thoughts or persistent pessimistic, fear-based thoughts. I'm referring to physical signals, like hunger, fullness, cravings, fatigue, bloating, headache, insomnia, and irritability. And spiritual signals, like inspiration and passion, or meaninglessness, purposelessness, and apathy. When we pay attention to these signals, they can guide us in meeting our daily needs.

When you eat emotionally, it's as if you're saying one or more of the following:

> "I don't know how to read my signals; all I know is that I *feel* physically hungry."
>
> "I don't know what I feel and need."
>
> "I'm afraid that if I allow myself to feel my feelings, I'll be consumed by them and might lose control."
>
> "I'm aware of my signals; I know when I'm hungry or full, and I know what I feel and need, but I don't know what to *do* with these emotions or *how* to meet my needs. I eat because I feel powerless and hopeless."
>
> "I can't meet my needs *until* I lose twenty pounds, get a nose job, straighten my hair, earn more money, become an extrovert, and so on; I'm stuck."

So you use food to calm, soothe, comfort, and pleasure yourself, distract yourself from unpleasant emotional states and powerless thoughts, and fill up an inner emptiness.

No doubt your emotional eating has helped you cope daily with self-defeating thoughts and emotional states like anxiety and depression. But it isn't a very effective long-term strategy for meeting your needs and desires. Not only does it lead to weight gain and poor health but it also can never be a substitute for learned skills. And you won't learn more effective self-care skills by going on another diet! Without these skills, you'll tend to feel somewhat disconnected from yourself and others. Your emotions, thoughts, and behaviors can become easily imbalanced.

You Started Out Life in Touch with Your Signals

You began life as an intuitive little being keenly in touch with your most basic signals. When you were an infant, physical sensations like hunger and fullness signaled you to reach for or push away from your mother's breast. Early in life, feeding was associated with pleasure, soothing, and connection. Other bodily sensations, such as tension or discomfort, signaled you to cry out for support and cling for comfort. As an infant, you depended on your caregivers to fulfill your needs and supply nurturance. (I use the term *caregivers* to include parents, grandparents, aunts, uncles, siblings, and anyone else who had a significant influence on your development.)

As you grew, your mind, body, and spirit signals continued to inform you of your needs and to prompt you to seek care. Each phase of your development involved specific developmental needs and particular kinds of nurturance. Childhood is a time of dependency, and we call these needs "dependency needs." When our dependency needs are consistently met with appropriate nurturance, we acquire the developmental skills we need to care for ourselves throughout our lives.

Stop for a moment and reflect: Were your caregivers kind and empathic? Were they good listeners? Did it feel safe to express *all* your emotions? Were they patient and comforting when you were upset or discouraged? Did they know how to soothe and comfort you when you needed it? Did they help you identify and meet your needs? Was it okay to have personal boundaries? Did they set and enforce reasonable limits? Were you treated with fairness and respect? Did you feel loved and valued? Keep in mind that even well-intentioned caregivers can miss the mark. The goal here isn't to find fault and blame; rather, it's to understand what might have been missing and where your skill building may have gone off track.

It's our caregivers' job to provide us with an environment that meets our basic physical needs (food, clothing, shelter) and emotional needs. We need our caregivers to help us identify and name our emotions. We need them to allow us to feel and express all our emotions and help us tolerate and navigate challenging emotional states by soothing us and teaching us how to soothe ourselves. And we need them to help us identify and meet our needs. This requires an atmosphere of patience, warmth, empathy, and understanding. We need to experience acceptance, emotional availability, good attunement, fairness, and respect.

It's important that our caregivers model positive, hopeful thinking and help us replace any pessimistic, self-doubting, or fearful thoughts. And it's helpful when they regularly express joy, happiness, and even excitement so we know that these emotional states are also possible and acceptable.

When our caregivers allow us free emotional expression and help us meet our needs, we learn to trust our signals and the goodwill of others. In this loving atmosphere, we develop an inner sense of safety, security, and trust, as well as a feeling of worthiness. We naturally develop self-acceptance and self-love. We learn where we end and the world begins, and that it's okay to have personal boundaries. We learn that there will always be enough. Enough love, joy, and care; enough mature and wise mentoring and guidance; and *enough nourishment*. In this environment filled with "enough-ness," we learn the important skill of self-discipline. We learn how to set reasonable limits and delay gratification of our impulses, so that we can take the best care of ourselves and meet personal goals.

The kindness and goodwill of our caregivers fosters the formation of a solid sense of self and good self-esteem. We begin to establish our own unique identity as our caregivers encourage our growing autonomy. We are able to separate from them, having developed a capacity for intimacy with and love of ourselves and others and the ability to identify and meet our needs.

Somewhere You Lost Touch with Your Signals

You may have grown up in an environment where, for a variety of reasons, your basic physical and emotional needs were inadequately met. Your caregivers may not have had their basic needs adequately met and may have been incapable of meeting yours. Even well-meaning, loving caregivers can be excessively self-absorbed or needy and regularly distracted by their internal struggles. Yours may have had a physical or mental illness. Perhaps they were angry, anxious, depressed, controlling, dominating, hypercritical, indifferent, irritable, intimidating, overindulgent, overprotective, out of touch, full of rage, or shaming. And the list goes on.

When our caregivers are inconsistent or unpredictable, we adapt to this stress by becoming hyperalert. Perhaps they worked too many hours and had too many responsibilities, and you felt neglected and abandoned. Maybe you were forced to spend much of your precious childhood trying to cope with unpleasant emotional states, insecurity, and low self-esteem. Your emotions and needs were neglected, and you lost touch with these important internal signals.

It's easy to see *how* we can begin to use food for comfort, pleasure, and calming. Unlike our neglectful family environment and chaotic inner world, food is soothing, readily available, and predictable. Rather than acquiring necessary self-care skills, we end up with skill deficits, which unfortunately can have lifelong consequences. We grow up with an emotionally starved inner child running our lives.

Perhaps Insecurity Is All You've Ever Known

In your childhood, you may have had to maintain your guard against emotional or physical abuse. You probably never thought of this as abuse or trauma; after all, it was all you knew. But moderate or severe neglect of our developmental needs is traumatic and can have a lasting effect on our psychological development.

Abandonment, attack, betrayal, blame, neglect, rejection, and shame are all examples of trauma. Emotional trauma, like physical trauma, creates wounds and leaves scars. Trauma results in and forces us to cope with chronic unpleasant emotional states such as anxiety, depression, sadness, emptiness, hurt, loneliness, and guilt. These emotional states distort our perceptions of ourselves, others, and our behaviors.

The neglect and abuse we've suffered creates what John Bradshaw, author of *Homecoming*, calls "toxic shame: the feeling of being flawed and diminished and never measuring up." The shame we feel makes it difficult for us to embrace *both* our strengths and weaknesses and develop a healthy level of self-esteem and self-acceptance. We lack the self-esteem to stand up to peer pressure and unrealistic cultural standards, and we begin to compensate for our lack of self-worth by trying to control our appetites and bodies.

The effect on our development depends on the severity of these adverse influences, the presence of more positive counterbalancing influences, and our own constitutional makeup. Children differ in their sensitivity to stressors. Some tolerate major stressors, while others fall apart from minor stressors.

Whether we are aware of it or not, we enter adulthood with a basic sense of insecurity. It's all we've ever known. We have a hurt, sad, angry, anxious, lonely, wounded child within. We're forced to present to the world a false self, the one our caregivers required us to adopt. We've become disconnected from our authentic self.

Trauma Distorts Thoughts and Behavior

The traumas you may have experienced, whether they were mild or severe, have affected more than your emotional well-being; they've most likely distorted your thoughts and behaviors as well. Perhaps your thoughts tend to be fearful, critical, negative, judgmental, obsessive, and self-defeating. In addition to emotional eating, you may resort to ineffective behavior patterns such as avoidance, procrastination, people pleasing, and striving for perfection to cope with unpleasant emotions and negative thoughts. You may also use shopping, busyness, drama, gambling, sex, or even self-mutilation to distract yourself from the pain. All these addictive behavior patterns compensate for your lack of self-care skills, and they perpetuate the pain.

Your Personal Boundaries May Be Too Loose or Too Rigid

Personal boundaries are a sort of invisible psychological edge, or limit, that defines where we end and another person, or the world, begins. Just like the skin on your body, these boundaries are meant to protect you by allowing the good to flow in and by keeping the bad outside you. They keep you safe by signaling whether someone's behavior or energy feels friendly or inappropriate.

When our caregivers model firm yet flexible, healthy boundaries, we grow up with clear, healthy boundaries of our own. Caregivers with poor boundaries raise children with poor boundaries. If your boundaries tend to be too loose, you'll feel somewhat merged or enmeshed with others and their needs. You may have difficulty identifying and expressing your own needs and asking for support in meeting them. Perhaps you regularly say yes when you really want to say no. You might have difficulty tuning in to boundary invasions; perhaps you're overly trusting and gullible. Or maybe you have keen antennae and *do* pick up the signals, but you have difficulty trusting them and fear asserting yourself. When your boundaries are too rigid, you feel lonely and disconnected from others. You may long for intimacy but fear the engulfment that you associate with closeness.

You *Can* Learn These Skills and End Your Emotional Eating

It may be comforting to know that many of us, not only emotional eaters, are missing skills from childhood, and that this leads to emotional, cognitive, and behavioral imbalance. We may not overeat, but a loved one may feel we use alcohol, drugs, drama, sex, pornography, video games, or anger to excess. Maybe we spend money compulsively or gamble irresponsibly. We may be a workaholic or use busyness as our drug of choice.

Perhaps we're chronically late, we procrastinate, or we have excessive clutter. Maybe we battle depression or experience chronic anxiety and panic attacks. Our relationships may be strained; we may have few friends. Perhaps we have difficulty with motivation and discipline in many areas of our lives. We may feel dull and apathetic and find our lives lack meaning, passion, or purpose.

The five self-care skills that follow represent the skills everyone, not just emotional eaters, must master to experience a solid sense of self and lead a fulfilled life. These skills help us take the best care of ourselves. Reconnecting to your authentic self takes time and is a process. It will require some practice and patience on your part. The good news is that these are all skills you can acquire.

The Five Self-Care Skills

Most weight loss programs attempt to apply external solutions to internal problems. They focus on what and how much we eat and how much we exercise. Yet as I've mentioned, it's our inner world of emotions, thoughts, and needs that drive our behavior. In order to understand the behavior of emotional eating, we have to tune in to and explore our inner world.

Focusing on external solutions, such as fad diets or exercise routines, is like trying to solve the problem of a derailed or stalled train by giving it a new coat of paint and polishing its wheels. No matter how much paint or polish we apply, the train will remain stuck. We need to access the engine that drives the train so that we can accurately diagnose the problem. The five self-care skills that follow are the tools you will use to get your train back on track and running properly. They represent the developmental skills and inner support system that help you maintain balance.

Skill #1. Establish the habit of self-connection.
Skill #2. Catch and reframe self-defeating thoughts.
Skill #3. Soothe the small stuff; grieve the big stuff.
Skill #4. Create a state of enough-ness, then set nurturing limits.
Skill #5. Practice accepting and loving yourself unconditionally.

You'll need to turn inward for this part of the journey. For some, this will be the most challenging part of the whole process. Hopefully, it will be illuminating and exciting as you identify and resolve the pieces of your personal emotional-eating puzzle.

Here, in part 1 of this book, you'll discover

- how to connect with and handle your inner world of emotions and thoughts — and how to deal with highly reactive emotional states and powerless thinking;
- how to identify your needs and meet them;
- the self-soothing and self-nurturing skills you didn't acquire in childhood;
- the importance of grieving losses and disappointments;
- how to identify and work through old pain left over from childhood experiences;
- how to set appropriate limits with yourself;
- how to delay gratification so that you can pursue your goals;
- how to tighten or loosen your boundaries where appropriate;
- how to practice self-acceptance and self-love; and
- the importance of regularly acknowledging your gains and strengths.

Consistently practicing the five skills is a sign that you've successfully made the transition from a derailed, *hungry* grown-up child to a satisfied, *fulfilled*, and confident adult.

Throughout your journey into the inner world, see if you can access a voice inside yourself that says, "Okay, I will try this." This is your willingness. It takes a bit of surrender. If you notice resistance, that's okay. Allow it to be. Embrace it for now. Be gentle and patient with yourself.

When you're ready, this voice will surface. It may even be small, quiet, and timid, hesitant from years of feeling like a failure at weight loss and other achievements. But it will be there. Look for it. It is the voice of your sweet, scared, wonder-filled authentic self.

CHAPTER TWO

Skill #1. Establish the Habit of Self-Connection

When we sat down in my office and I asked *her* how she was *feeling*, Carol, a petite brunette in her midforties, began, as usual, to tell me how *everyone else* in her life was *doing*. Her boss was stressed out and yelling, her husband was overworking himself, the kids were misbehaving, and her mother was being demanding and intrusive. When I reiterated my concern for how *she* was *feeling*, she responded, "Who has time to feel? All I know is that I'm overeating and drinking too much alcohol."

I asked her if she took any time during the day to check in with herself, and she quickly responded, "No." She admitted that it wasn't just a matter of little free time. "I'm not really sure how to check in with myself, and I'm also afraid to go inside. What if I get really upset and can't pull myself together?"

I could understand Carol's fear of "going inside." She had experienced a considerable amount of emotional neglect, criticism, and shame as a child. She'd spent her childhood years trying to please her mother and survive emotional abuse. As the oldest child, she had been expected to care for her three other siblings and put her needs on hold. Now the "voices" in her head tended to be harsh and critical. Of course she didn't want to go inside.

Throughout her childhood, food was *the* major source of comfort and nurturance and the one thing she could share with her mother. In college, Carol discovered alcohol and found that it was a great social lubricant and a tranquilizer. Carol's mother was disconnected from her own internal world and often complained of migraines, backaches, and other ailments. She was incapable of helping Carol identify her emotions and meet her needs. Carol had never learned the important skill of self-connection.

What Does Self-Connection Mean?

Self-connection simply means that you go inside regularly and check in with *your* inner world of emotions, needs, and thoughts. You continually monitor your internal world. Just like a master mechanic, you listen for signals of distress and make the required adjustments to meet your needs and stay in emotional balance.

The primary cause of your emotional eating is your disconnection from yourself. You're cut off from your most basic signals, your emotions. You still experience unpleasant emotions such as anxiety, frustration, and loneliness, and your overeating is an attempt to soothe, comfort, and distract yourself from these emotional states. It's also an attempt to bring in more pleasure and fill up on something outside yourself.

Getting clear on what you *feel* is the first step in determining what you *need*. In this chapter, I'll show you how to identify, stay with, and express your emotions (rather than disconnect from them or act them out) and how to identify and meet your needs. I'll also show you how to form an alliance with the wisest part of yourself, the part that can provide comfort and can support you in meeting your needs. I think you'll be pleasantly surprised to find how truly easy it is to practice self-connection and how it can reduce your emotional eating immediately.

Self-Connection Begins with an Inner Conversation

Whether we're aware of it or not, we all engage daily in silent self-talk. We experience our self-talk as thoughts. We tend to have a running monologue, saying things to ourselves such as:

"I think I'll wash the dishes before I throw out the trash."

"I'm going to finish this chapter and then turn the light out."

"I want to remember to call Sam about the plan on Friday."

We also have internal conversations, such as:

"I shouldn't have any more ice cream. But it tastes so good. I'll just have a little more; I've had such a hard day. I deserve it. Well, I've already blown my diet for today, so might as well finish the carton."

"I sure feel lonely these days. I wish I had a loving partner to share my life with. Well, that'll probably never happen. It's just too hard to meet people in this city. I think I'll order a delicious pizza and pasta dinner and settle in for the night."

Where Do These Voices Come From?

As we grow and develop, we internalize the voices of our caregivers, extended family members, siblings, and mentors. After we spend years listening to these voices, they become automatic and habitual. We're often unaware of them. They represent our *thinking self*, the part of our personality that includes experience, knowledge, intellect, wisdom, rationality, morality, and logic. This is the part of our self that can drive and initiate action and make decisions. Our *thinking self* can be a supportive, caring, and kind Inner Nurturer, a helpful or destructive Inner Critic, or just a neutral adult voice, as in the monologue examples earlier.

Our *feeling self*, the childlike part of our personality, represents our intuitive, sensing, vulnerable, feelings-centered, spontaneous, pleasure-seeking, wonder-filled, imaginative, authentic, core being. We all have this playful, instinctual inner self, even though we may not be in touch with it. This is the part of our personality that does not change or age with time.

If the adult voices of our childhood were primarily warm, kind, encouraging, hopeful, loving, validating, soothing, and nurturing, we begin to develop a supportive voice within that can restore us to emotional balance when needed. As we mature into adulthood, this supportive voice becomes the voice of our Inner Nurturer, our main source of validation, approval, and reassurance.

This isn't to suggest that we're emotional islands and never desire feedback and encouragement or reassurance from others. But if we've developed this internal nurturing voice, we can turn within more often for the support and comfort we need.

If our caregivers were judgmental, critical, unkind, or shaming, the dominant voice inside our head will most likely be that of a harsh Inner Critic. By taking on our caregivers' critical voices, we adopt a distorted view of ourselves and others. This voice beats us up and leaves us feeling lonely and unworthy. This voice tells us that we are basically inadequate, never good enough. We enter adulthood with a sense of insecurity and low self-esteem. We regularly feel unworthy, inadequate, lonely, anxious, and depressed.

Disconnecting from your inner world is a natural way to stop the critical voices in your head. But when you disconnect, you abandon your authentic *feeling self* in the same way you were emotionally abandoned by your caregivers. And you fail to develop and strengthen your inner supportive voice.

When you disconnect from your emotions, you miss the opportunity to make contact with your authentic *feeling self*, the source of your creativity, passion, and inspiration. Your world can become dull and meaningless. You might experience this dullness as an inner emptiness, loneliness, restlessness, or low-level depression. Disconnection and emptiness fuel emotional eating.

If you don't take time to experience and appropriately express your emotions, they seep out in other ways. It actually takes a lot of physical and psychic energy to push them out of your awareness and stay in control. Repressed emotion wreaks havoc on your mind, body, and spirit and often shows up in chronic body pain and symptoms of disease.

It's essential that you stop this generational cycle of inner disconnection and abandonment by turning inward more often and forming a positive, lifelong, loving alliance between your *feeling self* and your supportive Inner Nurturer. As you strengthen this alliance, you'll notice how nourishing it feels and how painful, albeit familiar, it is to listen to the Inner Critic. Over time, you can reduce and eventually eliminate the harsh, shaming, destructive voice of the Inner Critic.

To help clients practice the skill of self-connection, I developed a process I call Inner Conversations. Having an Inner Conversation involves three simple, easy-to-use steps, and takes only a few minutes.

Inner Conversations

STEP 1.   Ask yourself, "How am I feeling in this moment?"

STEP 2.   Ask yourself, "What do I need?"

STEP 3.   Use your wise Inner Nurturer voice to reassure and comfort your *feeling self* and address your needs.

Practice Self-Connection Using Inner Conversations

Try engaging in an Inner Conversation if

+ YOU WANT TO USE DISTRACTIONS such as food, alcohol, drugs, shopping, working, sex, gambling, drama, television, Internet surfing, video games, busyness, or excessive sleeping;
+ YOU'RE EXPERIENCING UNPLEASANT EMOTIONS like sadness, anxiety, depression, anger, loneliness, fear, guilt, shame, helplessness, or hopelessness;
+ YOU FEEL NUMB, which may be experienced as emptiness, boredom, apathy, lack of motivation, or feeling blah, lost, or disconnected;
+ YOUR THOUGHTS ARE OBSESSIVE, such as when you're thinking about food, meals, body image, or weight too much; regularly recycling self-defeating, critical, judgmental thoughts; or worrying constantly about anything; or
+ YOU ENCOUNTER STRESSFUL SITUATIONS such as difficult people, relationship struggles, social encounters, losses, disappointments, financial hardship, or illness.

Step 1. "How Am I Feeling in This Moment?"

If during your childhood it wasn't safe to express your emotions, as it was not during Carol's childhood, you may be unsure of what you're feeling most of the time. Emotions are unfamiliar and uncomfortable territory, period. Or perhaps, unlike Carol, you find it fairly easy to identify your emotions but more challenging to stay with them. When you do allow yourself to feel your emotions, you get overwhelmed by, obsessed with, or even paralyzed by them.

In my twelve-week program, workshops, and groups, when we work on identifying and expressing emotions, participants often tell me things like:

> "I don't think I have many emotions; I feel numb most of the time."
> "I can only experience my emotions briefly; then they're gone."
> "I'm aware of my emotions, but what should I *do* with them?"

Let me assure you that we all have a full range of emotions, whether or not we're aware of them. In the beginning, you may have to take your best guess as to which emotions you're experiencing.

Think back: During your developmental years, were you encouraged to identify and name your emotions? Were you allowed to fully express *all* your emotions? When you did express them, were they truly heard and validated? If not, you either began to push them down and disconnect from them (repression) or you acted them out through temper tantrums, moodiness, defiant behaviors, and emotional eating.

Identifying Your Emotions

You'll need to pull away from your busy world for a few minutes in order to access your emotions. With practice, you'll be able to do this anytime, anywhere. Find a quiet space where you can be alone (even a bathroom stall will do). Take a few deep breaths. Quiet your mind. Ask the noisy thought-generating part of your mind, your *thinking self*, to be silent for now. It's best to sit upright; lying down often leads to falling asleep, a sneaky way to avoid emotions.

I suggest that at least in the beginning, you write down your Inner Conversations and spend some time experiencing your emotions. It's too easy to get distracted by other thoughts if you try to do this in your head. You can buy a journal specifically for this purpose, or you can just grab some paper and start writing. Start by asking yourself, "How am I feeling in this moment?" The terms for emotions are just single words, such as *worried*, *excited*, and so on. Begin identifying your emotions with "I feel..." statements. For example, "I *feel* worried" or "I *feel* excited." Use table 1, "Seven Core Emotions," to help identify as many emotions as possible.

You might experience conflicting emotions at the same time. After the breakup of a relationship, you might feel anger, sadness, *and* relief. Perhaps you feel the joy of being alone *and* feel lonely. When your best friend loses a lot of weight, you may feel happy for her *and* jealous. Just allow yourself to feel all your emotions, without *doing* anything and without judgment or criticism. Just notice them like an interested observer watching a parade go by.

You may find that you're limited in your emotional experience and tend to feel one main emotion. Perhaps, like Carol, you feel agitated or anxious whenever you're really sad, disappointed, lonely, or guilty. Some emotions are more energizing, and you may prefer to experience these emotions. Other emotions, such as sadness, hopelessness, and shame, are more deflating. In your childhood, was it okay to be sad but not angry? In my family, expressing anger toward my mother could lead to World War III. It was safer to stuff it down and avoid confrontation and more pain. This, however, led to hopelessness and recurrent bouts of depression.

In an attempt to be different from your caregivers, you may also try to cut yourself off from particular emotions they expressed. Maybe you made a decision in childhood *not* to be like your raging, angry father. You find yourself always suppressing your anger even if it means experiencing chronic headaches or poor treatment from others.

Table 1

Seven Core Emotions

Happy*	Afraid*	Hurt*	Guilty+	Angry*
Appreciative	Alarmed	Dejected	Bad	Agitated
Blissful	Apprehensive	Disappointed	Culpable	Annoyed
Calm	Avoidant	Discarded	Regretful	Antagonistic
Centered	Concerned	Insulted	Remorseful	Bitter
Comfortable	Defensive	Invisible	Responsible	Contemptuous
Compassionate	Distressed	Offended	Sheepish	Disdainful
Confident	Disturbed	Rejected	Wrong	Disgusted
Connected	Edgy	Unimportant		Enraged
Content	Frantic	Unwanted	**Ashamed+**	Envious
Delighted	Frightened			Exasperated
Ecstatic	Helpless		Confused	Fed Up
Encouraged	Hesitant	**Sad+**	Culpable	Frustrated
Energized	Insecure		Disgraced	Furious
Enthusiastic	Nervous	Blue	Dishonorable	Guarded
Excited	Overwhelmed	Dark	Embarrassed ·	Grumpy
Fulfilled	Panicked	Defeated	Exposed	Hostile
Glad	Paralyzed	Depressed	Foolish	Impatient
Grateful	Petrified	Despairing	Humiliated	Indifferent
Hopeful	Powerless	Despondent	Improper	Indignant
Inspired	Rattled	Disappointed	Mortified	Irate
Joyful	Restless	Discouraged	Ridiculous	Irked
Loving	Scared	Distressed	Self-Conscious	Irritated
Moved	Shaky	Down	Shocked	Jealous
Optimistic	Shocked	Empty	Unworthy	Mad
Peaceful	Startled	Gloomy	Visible	Outraged
Pleased	Suspicious	Grieving	Vulnerable	Peeved
Refreshed	Terrified	Hopeless		Perturbed
Safe	Uneasy	Irritable		Resentful
Satisfied	Vigilant	Miserable		Upset
Secure	Worried	Morose		Vengeful
Strong		Sorrowful		Vindictive
		Unhappy		
		Withdrawn		

* These emotions tend to be energizing, even though they may not be pleasant.
+ These emotions tend to be deflating.

Can you identify how different emotions feel in your body? I experience sadness as an ache in my chest. When I'm anxious, I feel hyped up or, sometimes, as if there are butterflies in my stomach. Anger feels like tension in my body or head, and with shame I get a sinking feeling. When I'm happy, I experience a calm, peaceful, or energized feeling. Is there a color you associate with different emotions? Perhaps you literally *see red* when you're angry, or the world looks dark when you're depressed. With practice, you'll be able to identify a full range of emotions by how they present themselves in your body.

Mistaking Thoughts for Feelings

We all have a tendency to move away from our emotions by focusing on our thoughts. See if you can differentiate between your thoughts and emotions. Tell your *thinking self* that you'll come back to the thoughts later. Stay present to your emotions by writing down what you feel and by focusing on the sensations in your body. If you've been used to cutting yourself off from your emotions, you may feel hyperconscious and self-absorbed. It may even be exhausting to feel so many emotions. Keep in mind that in order to become your own best caregiver, you need to pay attention to these basic signals. Staying with your emotions, for at least a few minutes — and longer, if possible — affords you the time to process and learn from them.

When Carol expressed her emotions, she hardly experienced them in her body, and she got stuck in her thoughts:

> "I *feel* lonely. I *think* John works too much and helps out around the house too little."
>
> "I *feel* agitated by my mother. I *think* she expects way too much from me."
>
> "I *feel* annoyed by the kids' whining and demanding. I *think* it's just too hard to work full-time and raise a family."

Practice going back to your emotions by saying to yourself, "Let's stay with the feelings." You can also ask yourself, "How *else* do I feel about this?" to access the full gamut of emotions.

When I gently suggested that Carol stay with her feelings and asked her how *else* she felt about the situation, she was able to access additional layers of emotion and truly *feel* her emotions:

Carol: I *feel* lonely. I *think* John works too much and helps out around the house too little.

Julie: Let's stay with the feelings. How else do you *feel* about that?

Carol: Hmm, I also *feel* angry and abandoned. And I *feel* sad! I *feel* the anger as a tension in my arms, chest, and neck, and I *feel* the sadness as an ache in my heart.

At this point in our conversation, Carol began to cry. Beneath the loneliness and anger was a deep sadness about her marriage that she rarely allowed herself to feel. She and John had become disconnected, and she feared he worked long hours in order to avoid her moods and the kids acting out. While Carol found it painful to feel this sadness, she also found it relieving. She felt a sense of hope come over her; perhaps she and John could work on reconnecting. She also felt calmer and could see that she would not need to turn to food at this point. She was eager to see what was underneath her constant irritation with her mother.

Carol: I *feel* agitated by my mother. I *think* she expects way too much from me.

Julie: Let's stay with the feelings. How else do you *feel* about that?

Carol: I *feel* guilty, and wow, again, I *feel* alone and sad. And there's that ache in my heart.

Carol was surprised to find that underneath the chronic agitation and guilt was loneliness and sadness regarding her relationship with her mother.

Carol: Even though I've always been close to my mother, our relationship has been challenging. I'm really sad that we've never had the kind of loving relationship I see other daughters have with their mothers.

As Carol cried and allowed herself to grieve for the relationship they never had, she noticed that a sense of relief and calmness came over her again. We continued on to see what was underneath her feelings about her children.

Carol: I *feel* annoyed by the kids' whining and demanding. I *think* it's just too hard to work full-time and raise a family.

Julie: Let's stay with the feelings. How else do you *feel* about that?

Carol: Of course, I *feel* guilty, disappointed in myself as a parent — and there it is again, I *feel* sad. I'm really disappointed that I scream and yell at my kids so much, and I'm sad because they deserve better. I don't want my relationship with them to end up like the relationship I have with my mother.

"I See Myself as Weak When I Allow Myself to Feel"

When Carol expressed her emotions, her Inner Critic was often the first voice on the scene, shaming her for being a sissy. If your caregivers, like Carol's, had a negative view of emotional expression, you'll need to separate yourself from their view and create your own new, informed perspective. If, on the other hand, their emotions were regularly out of control and you long ago decided never to be like them — and so stopped expressing your emotions — don't throw the baby out with the bathwater. It wasn't the emotions that were bad; it was that they didn't know how to handle them.

Experiencing and expressing emotions is a normal part of being human. You did it all the time as an infant and a small child. We never outgrow the need to feel and express our emotions. By expressing your emotions, you can release energy and tension and communicate your needs to others.

Rather than viewing yourself as weak or pathetic when you acknowledge and express your emotions, realize that your ability to feel and tolerate all of your emotions makes you emotionally stronger and physically healthier.

"What Do I Do When the Feelings Won't Go Away?"

Carol was concerned that certain feelings — like the sadness she felt about her childhood — would never go away. Some emotions, such as the deep sadness we feel from severe losses or the anger we feel from betrayal, may be with us for a long time. These same emotions may reveal unhealed wounds from childhood. For the sake of our emotional balance, it is important to set aside time, as often as needed, to grieve.

Grieving is not a onetime event; rather it's a natural and important process that we engage in throughout our lifetimes. If we haven't been allowed to fully grieve losses and disappointments as children, we'll need to learn how to use grieving to restore emotional balance. I discuss grieving further in skill #3, in chapter 4.

"What If I Feel Overwhelmed by My Emotions?"

This is probably a sign that you've been disconnected from them for a very long time. You've been using eating as a way to calm down and reduce your sense of being overwhelmed. It's also a sign that your soothing skills need sharpening. You may feel vulnerable and raw when emotions surface. Perhaps in addition to feeling overwhelmed, you feel panic and anxiety. You may need to take a break from experiencing your emotions during your journal work. Take a walk, listen to music, read, or engage in some other nourishing *nonfood* distraction that calms you. Then try to go back to experiencing the uncomfortable emotions, if you can.

Some people find it is just too overwhelming to allow emotions to surface, and they experience an impending sense of being out of control or losing control. Perhaps you feel disconnected from yourself or the world, a state called dissociation. You may feel this way when you're very depressed or very anxious. If you have experienced trauma in your childhood, accessing emotions may bring up unresolved wounds with which you are not equipped to cope. Try not to see it as a sign of weakness if you need assistance.

A professional psychotherapist can offer you expertise and empathy and help you move through your natural resistance to accessing old memories and experiencing unpleasant emotions. If you choose to try identifying and experiencing your emotions on your own, it would be best to have a nurturing friend available for added support.

"How Do I Stop Overreacting and Acting Out My Emotions?"

Carol had a tendency to lash out at family members when she was feeling overwhelmed, anxious, and emotionally undernourished. "I yell, scream, criticize, and blame, and then I cut myself off from them with physical withdrawal and silence." She had learned these behaviors from her mother.

By learning to identify, express, and share our emotions, we can stop acting them out on others. Often our repressed emotions show up in reactions that don't fit the crime — that is, our emotional reaction is too big in relation to the situation. Terri, another client, also had a tendency to act out her emotions.

Terri asked Jake, her boyfriend, "Do I look fat in this dress?" Jake lovingly and gently tried to be authentic, replying, "Well, it's not the most flattering for your figure." Terri *heard* her father's critical judgmental remarks from childhood: "You are too fat for that dress; it looks awful." She stormed out of the house and refused to talk to Jake for hours. Terri was acting out the sadness, hurt, and frustration she had experienced and pushed away so many times in her childhood. When it comes to her body image, Terri feels fragile and needs soothing and comforting words. Her repressed emotions caused by childhood wounds have created a high level of emotional reactivity in her, and she is often on high alert (a pattern called hypervigilance) for criticism and judgment.

Jake actually unconditionally accepts Terri's body, but she was not able to remember this during their exchange. Jake felt misunderstood, confused, and made wrong for his best attempt at being lovingly honest. Terri's reaction reminded him of how *he* often had felt misunderstood in his family of origin and "how I could never get it right." When he tries his best and Terri overreacts, he feels helpless and powerless. He doesn't know how to soothe and comfort himself or Terri.

In childhood our caregivers may have unintentionally wounded us by highlighting our flaws or character defects without helping us overcome, improve upon, or accept and embrace them. Both Jake and Terri were wounded by not being loved and cherished unconditionally — chubbiness, mistakes, and all. Both were made to feel helpless and hopeless without proper instruction on how to improve the situation — for Terri, how to unconditionally accept her body as is *and* how to slim down if that's what *she* wants; and for Jake, how to "get it right" the next time.

For both Jake and Terri, an incident like this represents an opportunity to get closer to each other and express and share their emotions. It is a chance for them to heal the wounds from childhood and stop acting them out on each other.

Letting Go of Other People's Pain

As a sensitive, caring person, Carol had a tendency to absorb other people's emotions. Without realizing it, she was absorbing her mother's sadness and emptiness. She noticed that even though she felt fine when she arrived, after spending time with her mother, that would change. Her mother rarely shared her feelings, and even though the two women generally had a pleasant time together, Carol, as an empathic being, would pick up and carry her mother's disowned sadness and emptiness. The low level of depression Carol then felt would later, unknown to her, fuel her emotional eating.

As Carol recognized and acknowledged to herself her mother's pain, she was able to stop accepting responsibility for what her mother left unexpressed. She realized that she was entitled to feel joy and was not responsible for her mother's sadness and emptiness. Whether or not her mother chose to share it with her, Carol could be caring and compassionate, knowing that it was not her pain. Carrying her mother's pain didn't serve Carol or her mother. She no longer needed to eat in response to *her mother's* pain.

When you identify your emotions, try to assess whether each one is truly your emotion or someone else's by asking yourself, "Is this some-one else's emotion?"

Sharing Your Emotions with Others

Expressing your emotions is a way to allow others into your internal world. It opens the door for intimacy. It's an opportunity for growth and learning in a relationship. And it's not without risk. Hopefully, you'll be heard and well received. This may make you feel more vulnerable. And it might create conflict. You could get hurt, dismissed, abandoned, rejected, or even attacked. On the flip side, you might feel overwhelmed and en-gulfed by the closeness created and may need to regulate your sharing until you're more comfortable.

The best way to express your emotions to others is with "I feel..." statements. These tend to lessen defensiveness on the part of the recipi-ent when you're sharing unpleasant emotions. You might be dying to tell your friend who cancels plans at the last minute, "*You* are so inconsiderate and selfish; *you* always cancel plans late." However, expressing yourself this way doesn't truly convey how *you feel*. "I *feel* hurt and unimportant when you cancel plans at the last minute" conveys to your friend how you feel and how her behavior affects you. Similarly, you convey your emotions when you state to a family member who constantly interrupts, "I *feel* unheard, dismissed, and devalued when you constantly interrupt me." "*You* are very rude, and *you* interrupt everyone" does not express how *you*, in particular, *feel* in response to this person's behavior. Rather, this statement is somewhat judgmental and aggressive and may be met with resistance.

When we use "I feel" statements, we express one-word emotions directly after we declare, "I *feel*." Be careful not to assert, "I *feel* that *you*..." Here too such a statement would move you away from expressing your emotions and into your critical, judgmental *thinking self*.

Carol was beginning to see how powerful a tool self-connection could be. By practicing the first step of an Inner Conversation, she was allow-ing herself to feel all of *her* emotions and was releasing the tension that regularly built up inside. She immediately felt more calm and relaxed, and from this peaceful place she was ready to address her needs. She was able to take a more honest look at her life without the immediate need to comfort herself with food.

Step 2. "What Do I Need?"

If you've spent years disconnecting from your emotions, you're most likely unaware of your needs much of the time. After years of not getting many of your needs met, or focusing exclusively on the needs of others, you've probably become out of touch with them.

Perhaps some of these comments and questions sound familiar:

"I haven't the faintest idea what I need."

"I know what my husband needs, what my parents need, and what my kids need. But my needs, what are those?"

"Is it okay at my age to want time alone, to need support and affection, to want to be heard?"

"I feel like I *need* to say no more often, but is that an acceptable need?"

"I fear that many of my needs are childlike: I want to be taken care of, rescued, hugged, soothed, and reassured."

"How do I know if a need is realistic, if it's something I can expect to have met?"

"I often know *what* I need, but I truly don't know *how* to meet many of my needs."

As an emotional eater you may have been raised in a family where your basic *emotional* needs were poorly met. Perhaps you were not regularly touched, held, comforted, or soothed. Your caregivers may have been unskilled or too preoccupied to provide consistent attention, listening, understanding, wisdom, and guidance. You may have received little approval, acceptance, or validation. Criticism, judgment, and shaming may have been the norm.

Each phase of our development involves specific developmental needs and particular kinds of nurturance. We call these needs "developmental dependency needs" because we must rely or depend on direct caregivers and extended family members, as well as on people like teachers, counselors, and nannies, to meet these needs. We have fairly specific needs at each stage of our development. Good mental health depends on getting the majority of our needs met in the appropriate period of life. Each phase builds on the successful completion of the previous phase.

If our emotional needs are poorly met when we are children, we don't learn to *trust* that others can and will meet some of our needs or *how* to meet many of our needs ourselves. This sets up in us a lifelong pattern of trying, often unconsciously, to get many of our dependency needs met from the outside or of giving up on our needs. We are hungry for validation, approval, and reassurance. We look outside ourselves to know if we are worthy and valuable. We regularly seek encouragement and support from others, even if it's merely in the form of a look or a nod. We may crave the physical reassurance of being held and hugged. At the same time, we may feel ashamed of these needs or unworthy and try to hide them from others.

It's as if we're seeking to be reparented by other people in our lives. Other adults are busy meeting their own needs and obligations. We risk draining and depleting others if we regularly need them to emotionally take care of us.

We're *starving* to have these needs met even if we're unaware of them or deny having them. And often when we get our needs met, it feels like it's not enough. The intense craving for someone to meet our needs may feel like physical hunger. Food is pleasurable and temporarily meets some of our needs, but it's not food we hunger for.

Identifying Your Needs

Any upset, agitation, or urge to disconnect from yourself and use distractions like food is the cue that you're experiencing distress and have unmet needs. After asking yourself, "How am I feeling in this moment?" continue on to step 2 and ask yourself, "What do I need?"

Table 2, "Stage-of-Life Emotional Needs," gives a breakdown of our emotional needs from infancy to old age. Keep in mind that each stage represents the period when a particular need becomes most predominant. Take a moment to review table 2. Which needs call out to you? Which ones are you longing to have met? Be careful not to judge yourself during the process of identifying needs. Anything you discover is acceptable and valid. You're not bad or wrong because you have unmet needs. It's all right to feel needy.

Carol continued with her Inner Conversations, addressing each situation separately and asking herself what she needed. Her Inner Conversation regarding the fact that her husband, John, worked too much and helped out around the house too little went like this:

Step 1: How am I feeling in this moment? I feel lonely, angry, abandoned, and sad.

Step 2: What do I need? I need him to help with household chores, and I'd like him to be interested in my day and want to hear about it. Is that too much to ask?

Julie (as Carol's Inner Nurturer): It's perfectly okay to have needs. And yes, it's reasonable to need John to take on a fair share of the chores and to take an interest in your day. That's what partnering is all about.

Here is Carol's Inner Conversation regarding her mother's expectations:

Step 1: How am I feeling in this moment? I feel guilty, alone, and sad.

Step 2: What do I need? Boy, this is a tough one. I guess I need her to back off of her demands and appreciate what I do for her. This sounds odd, I'm sure, but I need her to be happy. But I don't *think* she's going to change.

Julie (as Carol's Inner Nurturer): It's understandable that you want and need her to make fewer demands and show appreciation for all you do for her. And of course you want her to be happy — for her sake and yours. You've clearly identified what you need. Let's not worry, at this point in the process, about whether *she* will change or ever be happy; you really don't have control over that.

Table 2
Stage-of-Life Emotional Needs

INFANCY (0–9 MOS.)	TODDLERHOOD (9 MOS.–30 MOS.)	PRESCHOOL AGE (30 MOS.–5 YRS.)	SCHOOL AGE (5 YRS.–12 YRS.)
Comfort	Acceptance	Acknowledgment	Adventure
Consistency	Attention	Approval	Affiliation
Echoing	Autonomy	Celebration	Awareness
Holding	Boundaries / limits	Clarification	Choice
Kindness	Empathy	Companionship	Competency
Love / care	Encouragement	Creativity	Connection
Mirroring	Exploration	Fairness	Cooperation
Patience	Fantasy / play	Fun	Counsel
Regulation of	Free expression	Growth	Honesty
emotional arousal	Idealization	Guidance	Industry
Relief of distress	Listening	Purpose	Information
Safety	Mobility	Respect	Mastery
Soothing	Nurturance	Structure / order	Mystery
Tenderness	Protection	Validation	Role models
Touching	Reassurance	Wonder	Separation
Trust	Support	Worthiness	Stimulation
	Understanding		

ADOLESCENCE (13 YRS.–18 YRS.)	YOUNG ADULTHOOD (19 YRS.–34 YRS.)	ADULTHOOD (35 YRS.–75 YRS.)	OLD AGE (76+ YRS.)
Authenticity	Commitment	Appreciation	Completion
Experimentation	Community	Beauty / aesthetics	Consideration
Fidelity	Integrity	Contribution	Contentment
Freedom	Intimacy	Expansion	Wholeness
Independence	Joy	Extension	
Justice	Meaning	Forgiveness	
Sexual exploration	Passion	Generativity	
Space	Productivity	Significance	
Spirituality	Purpose	Silence	
Variety	Recreation		

As you gain skill at having Inner Conversations, you'll see that you can make all the changes needed to stay in balance, whether or not others shift.

Carol's Inner Conversation regarding the kids' whining and demanding behavior went as follows:

Step 1: How am I feeling in this moment? I feel guilty, disappointed in myself as a parent, and sad.

Step 2: What do I need? I need to feel less guilty and disappointed in myself as a parent. So I guess I *need* to carve out more quality time with my children. The truth is, I *want* to have more quality time with them. I know — I *need* connection with each of them. Yeah, that's it. I need to stop yelling at them and acting out my frustration on them. I need to take a little time before I get home, even just in the car, and relax and switch into "mommy mode." And I need to work fewer hours at my job.

Julie (as Carol's Inner Nurturer): That's great! You've really gotten clear on what you need *and want* regarding the kids. And you've even begun to address the solution.

Meeting Your Needs

When you identify a need, see if you can break it down further into an even more specific need. Ask yourself, what would it look like if this need were met? Or, what would it take to meet this need? Perhaps you've identified a need to feel more love in your life. What would it look like if this need were met? Would you receive more affection? More connection? More intimacy? If it's clear that you need more connection, what would it take to meet this need? More time on the phone with good friends, better listening from your spouse, or something else? If you want better listening from your spouse, try to be even more specific. For example: "I *need* John to take fifteen to twenty minutes a few nights per week and lovingly listen to me and reflect back to me what he hears rather than just saying *uh-huh*."

Perhaps you identify a need for more support. What does that mean?

More encouragement? More help with household chores? Which chores? The more specific you can be in identifying your needs, the easier it will be for you to meet them.

Once you identify a need, it may take some flexibility and creativity to meet it. It's often easier to identify and meet physical needs than emotional needs. This is the point where you will access your *thinking self* and come up with a few ways to meet each need. The more you let go of rigid expectations and black-and-white thinking, the more you'll open yourself up to finding a satisfying solution.

Let's say you identify the need for adventure and stimulation and would love to take a long, action-oriented vacation but don't have the time or budget to do so. Perhaps a train ride to a new and different location or a hike in an unexplored area could partially meet this need. Maybe you've identified the need to be touched more often but lack a friend or partner who might provide this. Getting a regular massage or snuggling with a favorite furry companion could temporarily meet this need while you focus on ways to bring affectionate people into your life.

When you've identified one, two, or even three possible ways to meet a need, it's time to commit to action. This is where intention and follow-through are important. Intention means that you *intend* to focus on this need. If you're not committed to meeting this need, you might sabotage your success.

Follow-through is needed to make sure you stick with your goal until it's met. It may take many attempts or additional time to meet a need. Choose baby steps that allow you to succeed at meeting the need. Big lofty plans can leave you feeling like a failure, concluding that "this need can't be met" or "I'm just not equipped to meet my own needs."

Some of the needs you identify may be needs that were not adequately met in infancy or early childhood. Perhaps you *crave* attention, soothing, comfort, reassurance, safety, security, approval, or validation. Maybe you long to be held and hugged. You may be yearning for protection and a relief from distress. This is perfectly okay. The alliance formed between your Inner Nurturer and *feeling self* will be the key to ultimately meeting these most basic needs and getting your developmental train back on track. You strengthen this alliance and the voice of your Inner Nurturer every time you turn within and practice your Inner Conversations. Over time, you'll find that your needs grow up and become more appropriate for your age.

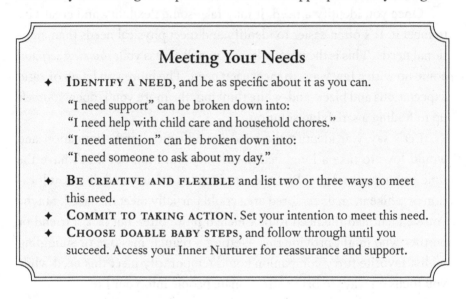

Meeting Your Needs

✦ IDENTIFY A NEED, and be as specific about it as you can.

"I need support" can be broken down into:
"I need help with child care and household chores."
"I need attention" can be broken down into:
"I need someone to ask about my day."

✦ BE CREATIVE AND FLEXIBLE and list two or three ways to meet this need.

✦ COMMIT TO TAKING ACTION. Set your intention to meet this need.

✦ CHOOSE DOABLE BABY STEPS, and follow through until you succeed. Access your Inner Nurturer for reassurance and support.

There will be times when your needs can't be easily or quickly met and you'll have to delay their gratification. Your closest friends may have moved away, and your need for companionship will be on hold until you can form new friendships. You may be newly divorced or out of a relationship, and your need for an intimate partnership may go unmet for a prolonged period. In the midst of a prolonged health crisis, you might not be able to get out and meet your need for fun and recreation.

Once again, these are times when a strong, soothing connection with your Inner Nurturer is important. This relationship will carry you through the rough times when you can't get your needs met by someone else. With your Inner Nurturer "by your side," you'll be better equipped to handle any sadness, disappointment, or frustration that arises because your needs cannot readily be met.

"It's Not Fair That I Didn't Get My Needs Met"

You're right! It isn't fair that many of your emotional needs were unmet when you were a child and that you now have to meet them yourself.

It's natural to feel sad or angry about this. You deserved to be loved and properly cared for. The sad reality is that in adulthood it's not possible to get your dependency needs routinely met from the outside.

Perhaps you don't feel equipped to meet your own needs. You're hoping to receive from other adults what you didn't receive as a child. You want *another* person to make you feel special, safe, and cared for. You want *someone else* to give you hope and tell you that you're okay and that everything will be just fine. You want *someone else* to be responsible for meeting many of your needs. You figure that if you get enough of your needs met from the outside, you'll *finally* feel complete and whole. Intellectually, your *thinking self* understands that you have to do this for yourself, but your *feeling self* isn't happy about it and is kicking and screaming.

Allow yourself to feel any emotions that might be surfacing when you read this — you're grieving the loss of a healthy, nourishing childhood. Grieving will help you release the pent-up emotion associated with disappointment and loss and prepare you for taking the best care of yourself *today*. I discuss grieving further in skill #3, in chapter 4.

As an adult, *you* are best equipped to identify and meet your own needs. No one can do this for you. This doesn't mean you won't get any needs met by others. It just means you'll be able, more often than not, to meet many of your needs yourself. This will free up your adult relationships to focus on adult needs such as intimacy, companionship, and recreation.

By practicing your Inner Conversations, you can learn to get clear on your needs. And with the support of your Inner Nurturer, you can find ways to meet your needs without turning to food or demanding too much from others.

Expressing Your Needs

There are times when you want to ask others for support, even though you can meet many of your needs on your own. Expressing your needs and asking for them to be met requires assertion and courage. It involves risk. You may fear rejection, anger, resentment, abandonment, shame, blame, and even unwanted responsibility for reciprocation. You might feel guilty and that you're burdening others. Perhaps it feels more comfortable to stay in control by giving and never receiving.

Do you feel selfish when you express your needs? Keep in mind that expressing your needs is a form of self-care, no more selfish than exercising or eating healthy foods. It's a way of acknowledging that you feel worthy enough to ask, that you live in this world with others and can trust and rely on them. You're making the statement "I have needs and they are important." It's also a way of respecting others by making your needs known and not expecting them to read your mind. You do, however, need to be respectful and recognize that others may not be able or willing to meet your stated needs. This doesn't mean you're unworthy or that your needs are not valid.

When you've denied your needs or disconnected from them for a long time, your attempts at expressing them and making requests can seem ungracious and demanding. If you've been passive about getting your needs met, when you finally do make requests you may sound angry, aggressive, and even cold. Maybe you deliver the request in an attacking, condescending way: "*You* haven't been helping out around this house; *you* need to be more helpful." Or "I'm sick and tired of being taken for granted; *you* need to consider my needs as well as your own." When you express your needs in this way, you may be met with confusion and defensiveness. Others are less likely to want to meet your needs. It can be helpful to practice expressing your needs and making requests by writing them in your journal before sharing them with others.

In order for our requests to be effective, we need to be respectful and considerate of the feelings and needs of others and deliver our requests with kindness, appreciation, and empathy. We begin by utilizing "*I feel…*" statements to express what we feel. We follow with "*I need…*" statements, making the need as specific as possible. Next, we move to appreciation, empathy, and respect for the other person's needs and feelings by utilizing an empathic "*I realize that…*" or "*I understand…*" statement that lets them know we've taken their needs as well as our own into consideration.

We end by asking for support in meeting our needs with an *"It would be great if you could..."* or *"I would appreciate if you would..."* statement. These last two steps are adapted from a process Laurel Mellin, author of *The Solution*, calls "the art of making requests."

Expressing Your Needs

✦ **BEGIN BY SHARING HOW YOU FEEL** with an *"I feel..."* statement.

✦ **STATE WHAT YOU NEED** with an *"I need..."* statement. Remember to be as specific as you can be.

✦ **EXPRESS YOUR RESPECT AND CONCERN** for the other person's needs with an empathic *"I realize that..."* or *"I understand that..."* statement.

✦ **MAKE A REQUEST** with an *"It would be great if you could..."* or *"I would appreciate it if you would..."* statement.

Carol decided to practice expressing her emotions and needs to her husband first, stating:

John, I *feel* dismissed and unheard when you try to move quickly past my emotions to finding solutions.

I need to just stay with my feelings.

I realize that you mean well and don't want me to feel sad or upset, and *I understand that* you care for me.

I would appreciate it if you would allow me time to process my feelings, and I'll let you know when I feel ready to look for solutions.

"I Feel Both Guilty and Needy When I Make a Request"

Uncomfortable emotions may surface when you ask to have your needs met. You may not be used to asking or to having someone say yes. My client Janet shared her experience and thoughts about asking her younger sister, Lana, for assistance:

I had never before asked my sister to watch my cats while I was away for a weekend — I always paid for a cat sitter. I noticed how I kept trying to minimize the amount she would have to help. I told her I would feed the cat Saturday morning before I left and Sunday night when I arrived home, and that if she could just stop by once or twice, it would be great. I realized that I felt guilty and not entitled to burden her with my responsibilities. *I also realized that by never asking, I got to feel like the sister who was always in control.* I never had to experience guilt, unworthiness, or dependency on another. By never asking, I kept distance between us. Lana helped me see that rather than feeling burdened, she felt like she was a part of my life.

We often experience a different set of emotions when we make changes in the way we handle our lives and interact with others. If we're not prepared for these new emotions, we can easily slip back into our old dysfunctional habits. Janet took a chance to ask for help, and she then felt some uncomfortable, unexpected emotions. She'll need to embrace these new emotions and see them as a sign of growth. As she practices making requests of others and lessening her tendency to be superindependent, she'll begin to experience worthiness, connectedness, and a healthy state of *inter*dependence. This will translate into more intimacy, less stress, and most important, less need to fill up on food.

Step 3. Use Your Wise Inner Nurturer Voice to Reassure and Comfort Your *Feeling Self* and Address Your Needs

If, like Carol, you feel you can't find within yourself a nurturing voice, see if you can model the voice of a kind, caring relative, mentor, therapist, or compassionate friend. You can also use the voice of a television or radio personality or public figure you admire. One client of mine used the voice of his father, who had long ago passed away. Another used the voice of her favorite television sitcom mom.

Most of us access a supportive voice within when we speak to small children or animals. Think about the voice you use when you greet a dog on the street or how you might speak to a small child lost in a grocery store. You would want the child to feel comfortable while you tried to help her. You would probably use a very soft, comforting voice. That's the voice! This voice may not be well developed if you haven't practiced it very often, but it's there.

"I Feel Silly and Awkward"

Clients often tell me they feel silly talking to themselves in this way. We often feel awkward when we learn something new. Think about how it felt when you first learned to ride a bicycle, play the piano, or speak a foreign language. With practice, it gets much more natural and comfortable. The important thing is to stick with it long enough to build emotional endurance and gain competency and mastery.

Over time, a shift you cannot now imagine will occur, and you will begin to feel comforted by your own voice and words. Your Inner Nurturer will be able to soothe and comfort you better than anyone you know or anything you could eat! Keep at it until you feel that shift.

When you're first learning to use Inner Conversations, you may find that they're only minimally comforting. They may feel more like work than comfort, and you may have to force yourself to practice them. The best way to become familiar with your inner world and strengthen your inner support system is to practice Inner Conversations daily. This doesn't have to take a lot of time. Think of it as a way to better get to know yourself. And keep in mind that you're *already* having conversations with yourself every day.

Carol was ready to push past her discomfort and complete her previously begun Inner Conversation concerning her mother, because she still felt disturbed regarding this issue. She was feeling calm about the situations with her husband and children and had a few ideas of how she could reconnect with them. She felt she was back in balance with respect to these issues and didn't need to go any further with these Inner Conversations.

If you *feel* back in balance after completing step 1 or step 2, you need not go any further. But if you have the time, it's always a good idea to practice using your Inner Nurturer voice in step 3.

Here's Carol's Inner Conversation regarding her mother's demands. Carol decided to try on the voice of an elder member of her church as her Inner Nurturer.

Step 1: How am I feeling in this moment? I feel agitated, guilty, alone, and sad.

Step 2: What do I need? I need my mother to stop making demands and appreciate what I do for her. I need her to be happy.

Step 3: Use my wise Inner Nurturer voice: It makes sense that you feel agitated when Mom constantly makes unreasonable demands. And she's not very gracious, so of course you feel unappreciated. Mom may not be willing or able to change her ways, so it's up to us to change. Let's lovingly tell her that we're just unable to be there for her all the time and that we hope she understands. I'll remind you that you don't need to feel guilty; it's not your job to meet all her needs and make her happy. In fact, you can't *make* her happy — happiness is an inside job. I know that you're sad that she isn't happy, but you can't change or fix that. You've already spent too much of your life trying.

Because this will most likely continue to be a challenging issue in Carol's life, she will have to practice her Inner Conversations many, many times. As she does this, many internal realizations and shifts will occur, and over time she will *feel* differently about the situation.

With a full Inner Conversation under her belt, Carol wanted to try one more regarding an area of her life that she knew would require change. It was clear to her that in order to create more quality time with family members, she would have to speak to her boss about cutting back her hours.

Here's Carol's Inner Conversation regarding her work situation:

Step 1: How am I feeling in this moment? I feel anxious, scared, and worried about telling my boss that I need to cut back. I also feel guilty that I'll be letting her and others down.

Step 2: What do I need? I need understanding, kindness, and some reassurance that it's okay to take care of myself and that I won't lose my job or upset others.

Step 3: Use my wise Inner Nurturer voice: It's certainly okay to feel the way you do. It's reasonable to want and need to cut back your hours at work. You have a husband and children who need you as well. Charlene [the boss] is a kind and caring person, and I'm sure she'll understand. In fact, she'll *have* to understand. You're not a superwoman, and you don't need to feel guilty for creating balance in your life. Let's discuss this with her first thing Monday morning.

THE INNER NURTURER'S JOB IS TO

+ help identify emotions, thoughts, and needs
+ validate emotions, thoughts, and needs
+ support
+ comfort and soothe
+ cheerlead
+ guide in meeting needs
+ provide hope
+ nurture (which includes setting limits)

THE INNER NURTURER MUST NOT BE

+ overly indulgent
+ overly permissive
+ childlike

"What If I Still Feel Like Eating after I Have an Inner Conversation?"

Set your goal to have an Inner Conversation *before* you eat, especially if you feel compelled to eat or want to binge. This means that you have the conversation when you have a strong urge to head to the drive-through, stop at the bakery, buy junk at the market, have seconds, or open the refrigerator again. Stay with your emotions for a while before moving on to your needs. If you have trouble identifying your needs, just repeat steps 1 and 3 until you feel more peaceful. From this calm place, it will be easier to identify your true *nonfood* needs and refrain from turning to food.

After having an Inner Conversation, you may still want to comfort yourself with food. Give yourself permission to use food for comfort afterward, if you need to. As you get more practice in using your Inner Nurturer voice, you'll be amazed at how quickly you can restore your *feeling self* to emotional balance and find nonfood ways to meet your needs. You'll feel more soothed and nourished internally, and the desire to overeat or binge will drop away over time.

CHAPTER THREE

Skill #2. Catch and Reframe Self-Defeating Thoughts

Have you ever *thought* about how powerful your thoughts really are and how quickly they can change your mood? Truthfully, how often does a thought or series of thoughts ruin a perfectly good day? How often do you grab something to eat to calm or soothe yourself because of anxious or depressive thoughts? If you're like the rest of us, you do it more often than you care to admit. Potentially scary news from the doctor's office or a notice from the IRS can instantly create anxious thoughts that are hard to shake. A misunderstanding with a coworker or rejection by a romantic interest might lead to agitated thoughts and an irritable mood. And the opposite is also true: an email from a dear friend or heartfelt appreciation from someone can create warm, fuzzy thoughts and an improved mood.

Researchers have demonstrated that the average person thinks a whopping twelve thousand or more thoughts per day. That's twelve thousand or more opportunities to feel good or bad! When the majority of our thoughts are positive, empowering, and optimistic, we *feel* good, "on top of the world," ready for the day, and as if we can accomplish anything. When our internal world is not so positive and is instead full of negative, critical, self-defeating thoughts, we *feel* bad — anxious, frustrated, depressed, hopeless, or powerless. These unpleasant emotions generated by our negative thoughts can quickly lead to an exaggerated desire for comfort and distraction. We may actually *feel* physically hungry, and food is a quick, albeit temporary, fix.

You may be routinely recycling self-defeating thoughts without realizing it. These thoughts might be about yourself, your body, your abilities, other people, the future, and even the past. Your mind chatter often begins first thing in the morning. You wake up, open your eyes, and realize what day it is, and here comes the first of the twelve thousand sound bites:

"There's too much to do today, and I'll never get through it."
"I'm tired, and it's going to be a long, hard day."
"I should have changed careers a long time ago; now it's too late."
"Life never seems to get any easier."

Then you catch your reflection in the mirror, and here come more sound bites:

"*Oh my God*, look how fat my stomach is...and I look so old!"
"What is going on with my skin? It looks terrible and blotchy."
"I'll never lose this weight; it's a hopeless battle."
"This outfit looks terrible, but nothing else fits; it'll have to do."

Your Inner Critic is on the job, loud and clear. No wonder you're already in a bad mood and hyperfocused on the pastries and donuts during the staff meeting.

Self-Defeating Thinking Leads to Emotional Eating

There was a point during my emotional-eating days when I realized that my overeating and recurring low moods were directly related to my thoughts. More specifically, they were a reaction (which my *feeling self* was having) to the evaluation and interpretation of situations and events (made by my *thinking self*). For example, while shopping for clothes, if I didn't like what I saw reflected back to me in a dressing room mirror, my overdeveloped Inner Critic would beat me up ruthlessly:

"I hate this body! It just doesn't fit well in clothes."

"I can't believe that with all the working out I do, I still look like this!"

"What's the use of trying to lose weight or stay in shape? I'll always have a body I don't like."

"It's just not fair that some people don't struggle with their weight and I have to watch everything I eat and exercise all the time."

I would leave the department store feeling frustrated, hopeless, and depressed. This would often lead to a binge and then more negative thoughts about myself. I might then spiral down and feel depressed for days or longer. I call this "doing depression" because it was actually within my control and caused by my own thinking (unlike depression caused by a biochemical imbalance). I began to understand that while I would never be able to control all the stressful situations or events in life, I could control the flood of negative, self-defeating thoughts and, as a result, my emotional states and my overeating. I realized that it was within my power to change my thoughts, and this gave me hope.

In order to change my thinking, I first had to become aware of *what* I was thinking. Whenever I wanted to grab comfort foods or overeat, and I was *feeling* sad, depressed, anxious, or hopeless, I pulled out my journal and wrote what I was *thinking* in addition to what I was *feeling*. I know this sounds tedious, but it was incredibly enlightening. I was amazed at how critical and judgmental my thoughts were. I realized that my overeating wasn't just a source of soothing and comfort; it was also a grand distraction from the powerlessness I felt in my life. It was easier to pleasure myself with food and then obsess about my eating and weight than to address the deeper underlying issues.

I could also see that some of my thoughts represented deeply held beliefs about myself, others, and the world. For example, in addition to the stream of negative body-image thoughts in the example I've just given you, there was a basic, core belief that I was not acceptable or lovable as is. I believed that I was not worthy of love unless I *looked* great. I was upset about my body because I believed that no one would love me the way I looked, and I would never be able to love myself. This belief was heavily reinforced by cultural messages — by magazine and television images everywhere of superthin women — that define attractiveness.

Our core beliefs feel like truths and can be challenging to alter. They are responsible for our continual insecurity, self-doubt, low moods, and constant desire for external validation and approval. They can produce painful emotional states and lead to ineffective behavioral patterns, such as overeating, people pleasing, perfectionism, avoidance, and isolation.

Aaron T. Beck, MD, author of *Cognitive Therapy and the Emotional Disorders*, suggests that these core beliefs can predispose us to excessive sadness and depression. A major technique of cognitive therapy is to make these beliefs explicit (we are often unaware of them) and then decide if they are effective or self-defeating. When clients learn to identify and challenge their thoughts and core beliefs, they often begin to feel better immediately.

Stinkin' Thinkin'

By recycling our self-defeating thoughts over and over again, we keep ourselves in constant emotional pain. The pioneers of cognitive therapy have identified many different kinds of distorted thought patterns. My own adaptation of these patterns includes emotional thinking, catastrophizing, black-and-white thinking, perfectionistic thinking, personalizing, overgeneralizing, exaggerating and minimizing, blaming, and obsessing and ruminating. In the following list, under each pattern, I've given examples of self-defeating thoughts and possible associated core beliefs.

Emotional Thinking

We're often unable to access logic and reason when we get stuck in our *feeling self*. Emotional states seem to become reality — if we experience something and "feel it," it must be the state of things.

Self-defeating thought:

"I just don't know how to handle this situation."

Possible core beliefs:

"I'm basically incompetent."

"I'm just not good at taking care of things."

"I need someone to take care of me."

"I'll never excel at anything."

"I'm worthless."

Self-defeating thought:

"I feel ashamed for not knowing such an obvious answer to the question."

Possible core beliefs:

"I'm basically stupid."

"I'm really a fraud; if they only knew."

"I can't do anything right."

Self-defeating thought:

"I feel invisible in this group."

Possible core beliefs:

"I'm basically boring and have nothing interesting to share."

"People aren't drawn to me, because I'm not interesting enough, stimulating enough, beautiful enough," and so on.

"People are drawn only to stimulating, attractive people."

We need to remind ourselves that when we're flooded with emotions and feeling overwhelmed or out of control, this is not a time to believe what we're thinking.

Catastrophizing

Were your caregivers regularly worried or anxious about upcoming events or possible outcomes? Did they frighten you with fear-based reminders, such as "be extra careful" or "it's not safe to…"? Perhaps they expressed catastrophic concerns regarding routine events such as taking the bus to school on a rainy day. The message you received was that the world is an unsafe, scary place. You were *not* taught the skills to cope with the difficult times, because your caregivers lacked these skills. You've learned to expect the worst and even to look for it, a state called hypervigilance.

Self-defeating thought:
"I'm experiencing some back pain; I'm afraid it might be a rare form of cancer."

Possible core beliefs:
"The worst situation will always happen."
"The outcome will be scary and painful."
"I won't be able to handle the pain. It will be terrible."
"I'll never feel safe and secure — it's impossible."

Self-defeating thought:
"My boss wants to see me in his office; I'm sure something awful will happen; I'll be reprimanded or, worse, fired."

Possible core beliefs:
"Bad things always happen to me."
"I'm powerless to change outcomes or improve my life."
"Finding good jobs is about luck, which I've never had."

Self-defeating thought:
"My mother is not answering her phone; I'm afraid something terrible has happened and she can't get to the phone."

Possible core beliefs:
"Something awful will happen and I won't be able to handle it."
"I will have to endure unending pain and hardship."
"Life will be all pain and no pleasure."

Cognitive therapy reminds us that certain words can create powerful negative emotions. Words like *awful* and *terrible*, and phrases like *it's impossible* or *I'm powerless*, can do just that. We feel worse when we think this way. We create an attitude of fear and resistance. We turn challenges and opportunities into catastrophes.

Black-and-White Thinking

Thinking in absolutes is a way of protecting ourselves by controlling the uncertainty of the world around us. Our thinking becomes polarized — we perceive things in extremes and see little gray area. Our world is clearly divided into good and bad, right and wrong, and this can lead to rigid thinking, the perspective that "this is the way it is." This applies to our eating habits as well: we are either out of control with our eating (overeating) or in control (dieting). This type of distorted thinking pattern stems from difficulties in early childhood, often because of an unpredictable and inconsistent caregiver.

Self-defeating thoughts:
"I ate a few cookies, which are not on my eating plan; I've blown
    my diet and might as well eat the whole box."
"I can't eat *any* nuts, dried fruit, bread, and so on."
"One bite and I'm out of control."

Possible core beliefs:
"I can't trust myself."
"I have to have perfect discipline or I'm out of control."
"I can't handle uncertainty, ambiguity, change, or imperfection."

Self-defeating thought:
"Walking for fifteen minutes, three times a week to start, is a waste
    of my time. I used to do the treadmill for forty-five minutes,
    five days a week."

Possible core beliefs:

"Anything less than perfect is not good enough."

"You either give something your all or don't do it."

"If I'm just mediocre, I'm not special, unique, *someone*."

Self-defeating thought:

"I've gained back a few pounds; I'm sure I'll gain it *all* back."

Possible core beliefs:

"A small setback always leads to failure."

"I can't trust myself to follow through."

"I have no control over anything."

By being willing to experience the "gray area" emotions, we can move toward developing more flexibility and spontaneity.

Perfectionistic Thinking

Do you beat yourself up emotionally for perceived mistakes, flaws, or failures? This type of thinking is a form of black-and-white thinking that often develops in response to controlling and demanding caregivers. It stems from the core belief "If I'm perfect and do everything that pleases Mom/Dad, then I'll get the love (care, approval, validation...) I need." Many emotional eaters are "good girls" and "good boys" who attempt to be perfect in many areas of their lives. If they can control their behavior, which includes eating, then they will not have to experience any unpleasant emotions regarding their bodies or selves. Examples of perfectionistic thinking:

"I blew my diet and it's only breakfast; the whole day is ruined."

"I feel really ashamed when I make a mistake that someone notices."

"Unless everything I do is near perfect, I feel like a failure."

"If my house is messy, I'm a horrible homemaker."

"I've been progressing nicely with my exercise routine; this injury will ruin all my good progress."

This style of thinking stems from a lack of unconditional acceptance in childhood. The dominant voice in your head is that of a harsh, shaming Inner Critic. Learning to challenge your unrealistic expectations will help you replace these thoughts with more realistic ones. Practicing your Inner Conversations and the unconditionally accepting voice of your Inner Nurturer will help you develop tolerance for and acceptance of your imperfections and inevitable errors.

Personalizing

When you feel rejected, dismissed, neglected, or even attacked, it certainly *seems* personal. After all, the other person or group is doing it to *you*. And yet it's not really about you at all. The way other people treat you says more about them and their problems than you. Let's say you go on a date and have a seemingly nice time, and the other person never calls you again. You can *personalize* the seeming rejection by saying to yourself, "I'm sure I'm not attractive enough for this person," or, "I'm sure I wasn't a stimulating conversationalist." However, it may be that neither statement is true. The person may have found you attractive and stimulating and may be intimidated by attractive, stimulating people. Or perhaps he or she found you very interesting and attractive but met someone else at the same time.

My client Shana personalizes other people's bad behavior. If someone is rude to her, she wonders why the person doesn't like her or what she might have done to warrant rudeness. If a somewhat self-absorbed friend fails to return a phone call or invite her to join a social event, she concludes that *she*, Shana, is not popular and well liked.

Possible core beliefs:
"I'm responsible, in some way, for other people's behavior."
"If someone is angry or upset with me or rude to me, there must be something I've done to cause it."
"If someone rejects me in some way, there must be something undesirable *about me*."

"People should treat me in the same considerate manner I treat them."

This type of thinking pattern generally results from a childhood in which we have experienced criticism, rejection, blame, shame, and even attack. Children are inherently narcissistic and see themselves as the center of the universe. "If Dad is always angry and yelling, I must have caused it." "Mom would stop drinking if I were a better daughter."

By becoming aware of your tendency to personalize other people's behavior, you can stop blaming and shaming yourself and others. There are many possible interpretations of situations and the behavior of others, and it's important to consider these before concluding that it's all about you, or that it's your fault. Your tendency to personalize may highlight a need to adjust your expectations of others.

Overgeneralizing

When you make sweeping generalizations out of single events or a series of events, or use words that convey extremes, like *always, never, all, forever, no one, everyone*, you are overgeneralizing.

Self-defeating thoughts:
"We've tried to get pregnant for six months; I'm sure I will never conceive — I'm *always* the one who misses out."
"I know this slowdown will last *forever* and I'll *never* be able to grow my business and earn a consistent income."
"I made a mistake with that client; I'm just no good at this business."
"It will *always* be a struggle for me to lose weight."

Possible core beliefs:
"I'm powerless to change the circumstances of my life."
"I don't deserve a happy life."
"Patterns represent facts that are near impossible to change."
"There is some law or form of destiny that controls my chances for happiness."

Similar to black-and-white thinking, this pattern distorts your thinking by the use of words that convey extremes. This type of thinking tends to develop in households where caregivers are critical and shaming and fail to provide hope for challenging situations.

Exaggerating and Minimizing

Do you have a tendency to exaggerate your flaws and failures and minimize your strengths, abilities, and lovely qualities? Emotional eaters tend to focus on their perceived flaws often to the exclusion of other, more positive traits. This pattern represents a form of tunnel vision and, as with other patterns, typically occurs because we were criticized and ridiculed as children and we have a fear of being found defective.

You're using this distorted thought pattern when, for example, you gain back a few pounds after a large weight loss and you're convinced that "I will gain all the weight back that I lost and once again will fail at weight loss." When you do this, you are minimizing the wonderful effort you have applied to losing the weight, and you are forgetting to recognize your achievements.

We often minimize the compliments we receive in a day or a week and exaggerate or magnify our flaws or any critical commentary we've received. Someone comments on what a great job you've done, and you say:

"Yes, but I could have done much better."

Someone tells you that your hair looks great, and you say:

"Thanks, but it's dirty and looks a lot better freshly washed."

Your employer writes in your annual evaluation that your performance overall has been very good and that he sees room for improvement in your organizational skills. You conclude:

"I'm terrible at organization; I'll never be promoted in this company."

You're exaggerating the critical commentary and minimizing the overall positive tone of the evaluation.

Possible core beliefs:

"I'm unlovable, worthless, and bad unless I do it all right."

"I'm basically defective."

"Things are rarely perfect, and when they are, it never lasts."

These thinking patterns can leave you feeling insecure, frustrated, never good enough, and hungry! By paying attention to your thoughts, you can learn to stop magnifying your faults and errors and discounting your accomplishments and successes. Start today to give yourself credit where credit is due.

Blaming

This distorted thinking pattern, typically modeled by blaming caregivers, is a way to avoid responsibility for your life. It distracts you from feeling your own pain as your focus becomes external.

Self-defeating thoughts:

"I can't lose weight, because there's too much junk food around."

"I can't find a better job, because it's all about who you know."

"I'm unfulfilled in my marriage because my husband works too much and is never home."

Possible core beliefs:

"I'm not responsible for my pain; I didn't cause it."

"I can't change the conditions of my life."

"I'm helpless and powerless to change my life."

Stopping the blame game is the first step in becoming real with yourself and facing your own pain. You can change or accept the circumstances of your life, but first you must be willing to take full responsibility for your life.

Obsessing and Ruminating

Our thinking is considered obsessive when it's dominated by a persistent idea, image, or desire. Perhaps you can't stop thinking about germs, your thighs rubbing, or the flabby skin under your chin and what you're going to do about it. Have you ever replayed a situation or an incident over and over again, analyzing it and reanalyzing it, trying to sort out who did or said what and who was at fault?

There are certainly times when we need to replay a situation in order to assign responsibility and learn from it. When this process becomes obsessive, we call it *rumination*, named after ruminant animals, such as cattle and sheep, which chew and rechew their partially digested, regurgitated food. You may have learned this type of thinking because your caregivers modeled it, or you may have developed it in an attempt to make sense of constant criticism and humiliation.

There are many well-known techniques to handle obsessive thoughts. There are thought-stopping techniques, such as snapping a rubber band worn on your wrist or ringing a loud bell, every time you ruminate. You can also carry around a piece of paper with the word STOP on it in big letters. Distracting techniques, such as reading a book or playing a musical instrument, shift your attention and concentration elsewhere. A more lasting solution is to challenge and dispute these disturbing thoughts.

Replacing Self-Defeating Thoughts

Our self-defeating thoughts and beliefs are usually triggered by situations that cause distress: disappointment, loss, hurt, fear, rejection, criticism, shame, vulnerability, and exposure. I've developed a process I call "Catch and Reframe" to help clients identify their irrational thoughts and core beliefs and replace them with more objective, nonjudgmental, energizing thoughts. The process involves two simple, easy-to-practice steps.

> ## Catch and Reframe
>
> **STEP 1.** **CATCH** your thoughts about any situation causing distress. Write down what you're thinking and feeling. Pick the most troubling thought to work on.
>
> **STEP 2.** **REFRAME** this thought or belief with a neutral or energizing new thought that feels equally true.

It may seem like an impossible task to change deeply ingrained beliefs you've held for a lifetime. It will definitely take some dedicated time and attention. Remind yourself that it takes a lot of energy each day to manage sadness, emptiness, anxiety, depression, and hopelessness. It would be a better use of your time to work on shifting your thoughts.

Step 1: Catch your thoughts about any situation causing distress. Write down what you're thinking and feeling. Pick the most troubling thought to work on.

Stop for a moment when you're experiencing unpleasant emotions or before you grab something to eat when you're not hungry, choose unhealthy comfort food when you *are* hungry, or eat beyond fullness. See if you can identify something that's bothering you and what you're thinking and feeling about it. If it isn't clear, take your best guess.

Don't shortchange yourself by trying to do this step in your head. You'll need to be focused when you do this work. Begin by writing down any and all things you're thinking and feeling. Don't edit or censor yourself.

Select the most painful thought about *yourself* or *your* life and how *you* feel, and focus on it. Don't worry about whether a thought is a core belief or not. Just write down all your thoughts. The core beliefs will become evident to you as you write them — these are beliefs you have held for a very long time.

EXAMPLE 1

Situation causing distress:
Sherrie just spent the afternoon with a good friend who lost a lot
    of weight and talked about it nonstop.

Sherrie's thoughts about herself:
"I'll never lose my excess weight."
"I'm not a motivated or disciplined person; I guess I'm lazy and I
    always take the path of least resistance."
"I don't like to exercise as much as she does, so it will be harder
    for me to lose the weight."
"My body would never look as good as hers even if I lost the
    weight."
"I don't have the support system she has, and I never will."
"She's younger than me; I should have lost the weight at her age."
"I'm a big, fat failure."

Sherrie's feelings:
Drained, invisible, jealous, defeated, inadequate, sad, hopeless,
    powerless, and depressed.

Sherrie's most painful thought:
"I'm not a motivated or disciplined person; I guess I'm lazy and I
    always take the path of least resistance."

This self-defeating thought happens to be a very painful, long-held
core belief. As a child, Sherrie was compared to her slim, highly driven
sister. Her father often labeled her as lazy. This label has stuck with her, in
her head, for a lifetime. I asked Sherrie to stop and *feel the pain* associated
with this belief. She shared that she *felt* depressed and hopeless when she
thought of herself in this way.

EXAMPLE 2

Situation causing distress:
Dana notices the clutter around her home and the piles of work
    she needs to address.

Dana's thoughts about herself:

"This is overwhelming for me; there's just too much to do."

"I can't get through all this."

"I need someone else to help me take care of all this."

"I'm missing something other people have."

Dana's feelings:

Overwhelmed, anxious, agitated, restless, frustrated, helpless, unmotivated, disappointed, and sad.

Dana's most painful thought:

"I'm missing something other people have."

Dana started to cry when she stated this core belief. It felt like a secret she had been carrying since childhood. She had been raised by her grandmother, and she could still hear her grandmother's voice telling her that she couldn't do anything right.

EXAMPLE 3

Situation causing distress:

Karen attended a weekend weight-loss retreat and felt excluded
and rejected by some of the women.

Karen's thoughts about herself:

"I'm never part of the 'in' crowd."

"It's unfair that some larger women rejected me because I'm
smaller; my weight problem is just as challenging as theirs."

"I put out a lot of effort to be friendly, and it always goes unno-
ticed."

"I never feel like I fit in anywhere."

Karen's feelings:

Angry, rejected, hurt, sad, defeated, discouraged, hopeless, resentful, and bitter.

Karen's most painful thought:

"I never feel like I fit in anywhere."

As Karen read this thought out loud, she could feel an ache deep in her chest. It represented a lifetime's worth of anger and sadness stuffed down and numbed out with nightly binges of ice cream and cookies. She longed to feel like she belonged, somewhere.

Step 2: Reframe this thought or belief with a neutral or energizing new thought that feels equally true.

Once you've identified your self-defeating thoughts and core beliefs, it's time to replace them with empowering new thoughts. I always like to start with any core beliefs because once these have been shifted, it's often easier to release associated negative thoughts.

Creating energizing replacement thoughts is often the most challenging (and exciting!) part of this whole process. You've been recycling some of your self-defeating thoughts for decades or longer. New thoughts don't *feel* true right away, even if intellectually you know them to be true. Initially, new replacement thoughts may not be comforting. Be patient with this process. Practice writing and verbalizing your new energizing, reframed thoughts daily. It will pay off.

EXAMPLE I

Sherrie's most painful thought:
"I'm not a motivated or disciplined person; I guess I'm lazy and I always take the path of least resistance."

Sherrie's reframes:
"I'm not really lazy — I procrastinate because I feel anxious, overwhelmed, and discouraged."
"I feel more motivated to exercise and eat right when I'm patient with myself and praise myself for small steps."
"When I adjust my expectations about the pace of weight loss and set realistic goals, I *can* accomplish them."
"I feel more motivated when I remind myself that I'm not in competition with anyone."

Example 2

Dana's most painful thought:

"I'm missing something other people have."

Dana's reframes:

"I *am* capable of making a realistic to-do list and accomplishing it."

"I'm learning how to go slow, practice patience, and break down large, daunting projects into small, doable tasks."

"My procrastination is related to my perfectionism; as I release my desire for things to be perfect or to go at a faster pace, I complete tasks in a more timely fashion."

"As I clear out my clutter, I can put systems in place that will help me continue to keep things orderly."

"The fact that I'm missing some life skills doesn't make me inherently defective or deficient."

Example 3

Karen's most painful thought:

"I never feel like I fit in anywhere."

Karen's reframes:

"I *can* find places where people are similar to me and more welcoming."

"I don't have to work hard to be liked or included."

"I am a likable person, *as is*."

"As I practice loving myself, others are attracted to me."

"Self-love and -respect are very attractive."

Suggestions for Creating Energizing Reframes

Once you come up with new, more energizing, reframes, you can use them repeatedly to restore yourself to sane thinking and an uplifted emotional state. This is a surefire way to interrupt your emotional eating. Here are a few suggestions to help you get started:

1. Keep them simple, short, and in the present tense. Avoid statements such as "When I ..." or "Sometime in the future, I will ..." You are living life in *this* moment, not waiting for your life to begin. This is not a dress rehearsal.

2. Make them unconditional. Avoid statements such as "If this happens, then ..." Try on phrases like "I am ..." or "I can ..."

3. Phrase them in a positive way, affirming what you are doing rather than what you are not doing. Rather than "I do not say negative things to myself anymore," try statements like "I choose to say only loving, supportive comments to myself."

4. If you can't think of an energizing, positive thought, try on a neutral, nonjudgmental thought. "My hair is thin, flat, and unattractive" can be replaced by "My hair color is a good match for my skin tone."

5. If you can't find any reframe that works, see if there is a deeply held core belief underneath the thought you are working on. Ask yourself, "What does this thought mean to me?" "My hair is thin, flat, and unattractive" may actually represent this core belief: "No one will love me with imperfections." Work on creating a reframe for the core belief. For example: "As *I* practice loving myself with my imperfections, I am attracting people capable of loving me *as is*."

6. Make your reframes self- and life-affirming. Try on statements like "I'm proud of ...," "I deserve ... ," or I'm fortunate that ..."

7. Think of something you would say to a friend or loved one to comfort her and help her see the situation in a new light.

8. Pretend you are talking to a young child. Many of the critical things you've been saying to yourself you would never say to a young child.

9. Try gratitude statements to help you value what you have. "I hate my ugly feet; they're twisted from years of wearing high heels" can be reframed into "I am grateful that my feet are healthy and sturdy and get me where I want to go."

10. Act as if you believe these new thoughts, until your feelings catch

up with your wisdom. See if you can temporarily experience a new thought as a truth you'd *like* to believe. For just a moment, try it on, suspend your "voice of reality," your doubts, and your "yes, buts" and allow yourself to experience the possibility. For a moment, adopt a childlike imagination where anything is possible. Practice your new thought often, using it whenever the old self-defeating thought or core belief surfaces.

When you're short on time, try to come up with a quick neutral or uplifting thought. Thoughts that restore hope, possibility, and optimism lead to more effective, productive action.

Here are a few more examples of energizing reframes:

Self-defeating thought:
"I'll never find a partner; I'm just too old."

Core belief:
"Men only want young, beautiful women."

Energizing reframes:
"I'm sure there are emotionally mature men who prefer someone
    closer to their own age."
"There are many single men available today."
"I only need to meet one man."
"My self-love is very attractive."
"I am worthy of love."

Self-defeating thought:
"I can't lose this weight, because there isn't enough time to focus
    on myself, to exercise, and to eat right."

Core belief:
"I can't take care of so many things at once."

Energizing reframes:
"I'm worthy of time and attention."
"I can make a few small dietary changes that support my health
    and well-being."

"I'm willing to take the stairs more often and to park farther from my destination."

"Small, baby-step changes are a good start."

"I'm capable of setting priorities and balancing the many demands of my life."

Self-defeating thought:

"It's hopeless — I'll never have thin, firm thighs."

Core beliefs:

"I can't love and accept myself *as is*."

"No one else will love and accept me this way."

Energizing reframes:

"My life is about so much more than the shape or firmness of my thighs."

"In this moment, I choose to practice unconditionally accepting my body as it is."

"I am much more than my thighs; I have many wonderful attributes."

"I'm doing my best to firm and tone my thighs; that's all I can do."

"In this moment, I choose to focus on my gratitude for all that my legs have carried me through in life."

Self-defeating thought:

"If I have one piece of cake, I'll blow my diet. I have to stick to a rigid eating plan or I'm out of control."

Core belief:

"I can't trust myself and need to impose rigid limits on myself."

Energizing reframes:

"I can choose to stop eating after one piece of cake and accept and tolerate the discomfort of wanting more."

"I'm willing to be uncomfortable in order to reach my goals."

"In this moment, I'm willing to be present to my emotions."

"I take good care of my *feeling self* by allowing her to have treats and by setting realistic limits."

Self-defeating thought:
"I never stick with anything; I'm terrible at follow-through."

Core belief:
"I just don't have patience, perseverance, or endurance."

Energizing reframes:
"In this moment, I choose to practice patience."
"As I relax and apply myself, I access my willingness to continue with this task."
"As I remind myself that I *can* endure, I'm able to stay with this challenging project."
"I *can* tolerate the frustration this project involves and see it through to completion."
"I'm capable of delaying gratification."
"I give myself the gifts of time, exploration, and patience to allow my talents to surface."

When You Need More Skill Building

It's possible that all you need in order to give your emotional eating the boot is self-connection — identifying your emotions, needs, and thoughts; and then accessing an inner nourishing voice to help you meet your needs and reframe any self-defeating thoughts. But if you've experienced considerable loss, disappointment, or trauma in your life, these first two skills may not be enough to restore emotional balance. If you're getting stuck in unpleasant emotional states and having difficulty reframing self-defeating thoughts, the next skill will be an invaluable addition to your bag of tools.

CHAPTER FOUR

Skill #3. Soothe the Small Stuff; Grieve the Big Stuff

C an you remember the disappointment you felt when you were young and you performed poorly in a swim competition or spelling bee? Or that it felt catastrophic to misplace or lose your favorite doll or some other object of your affection? Did you experience a difficult adjustment period when you lost friends because of a move or change in school? Losses and disappointments are an inevitable and necessary part of life. They begin as early as infancy when, for example, we lose center stage because our parents have another child and we have to share their love. Minor losses and disappointments offer us the opportunity to grow by learning how to express our emotions, accept the loss, take a lesson if there is one, let go, and move on.

Unfortunately, significant losses and traumatic experiences too occur in childhood. If we are raised in a family with patient and caring adults, our painful experiences and losses are acknowledged. Caregivers are available and responsive; and whether the losses are minor or significant, they are registered. Our caregivers help us manage the unpleasant, conflicting emotions we're experiencing. They allow us the time we need to grieve, and they assist us in adapting to and assimilating the loss. They use their words, tone, and behaviors to calm and soothe us and to provide comfort. They apply the equivalent of a healing balm to our emotional pain.

With proper modeling, we naturally develop an inner voice that is soothing, calming, and reassuring. Our ability to self-soothe is at the core of separating from our caregivers and establishing our independence. It means we can effectively cope with situations that cause distress and take actions to restore emotional balance.

Self-soothing is a skill you were supposed to learn in childhood. If your caregivers never learned to soothe themselves, they would not have been able to model and teach you this skill. Without this skill, you may get stuck in unpleasant emotional states and have no way to process and resolve conflicting emotions. The feelings are intense and unrelenting, so you cut yourself off from them and stuff them down, or you act them out.

Grieving is the process of accessing and expressing the full gamut of emotions associated with loss and disappointment. This process may include, in addition to sorrow, emotions such as shock, anger, rage, shame, fear, guilt, remorse, hopelessness, and powerlessness. Just like eating, grieving is innate and spontaneous. When empathic caregivers model and encourage grieving, it becomes part of our bag of tools for restoring emotional balance.

In many cases, whether intentionally or not, our caregivers were the source of our chronic painful experiences. When we are raised in dysfunctional family environments, we don't learn how to soothe ourselves or constructively mourn our losses. In this chapter, I'll show you how to self-soothe and grieve. With this skill set under your belt, you'll be able to handle just about anything life throws your way.

Looking for Soothing in All the Wrong Places

When we are raised in an environment deficient in nurturance and soothing, we unconsciously adopt defense mechanisms to help us cope with emotional pain. These mechanisms represent the lengths we go to in order to push our painful memories out of awareness. You may notice that you have trouble remembering painful childhood events (this is an act of repression). Perhaps when you're distressed, you have a long-standing pattern of disconnecting from yourself and going numb (dissociation). Or maybe you distract yourself from the pain you feel by minimizing it (rationalization or intellectualization): "I'm sure they did the best they could, given the situation." "Hasn't everyone had challenges?" "It's the past; I'm over it."

When we haven't internalized a kind, soothing voice, we continue to try to get our need for soothing met from the outside. As adolescents and young adults, we may still try to get soothing from our original caregivers, especially if they were able to soothe us some of the time. This approach generally leads to frustration and disappointment as caregivers reopen old wounds by failing once again to provide consistent, reliable comfort.

As adults, we may attempt to get our need for soothing met by those closest to us — our spouses, partners, close friends, mentors, and even our children. This often places too much burden on others. Some of us compensate for our unmet soothing needs and lack of self-soothing skills by becoming superindependent — unconsciously disowning these needs, denying we have any need for soothing. Denying our need for soothing does not, however, get rid of it, and we may attempt to overcontrol our lives so as to minimize uncertainty and discomfort. One way or the other, we end up expecting too much from others or too much from ourselves. And we fail to learn the important skill of self-soothing.

Self-Soothing Begins with an Inner Conversation

Self-soothing is the way we restore balance when we're upset or distressed, and we do it on an as-needed basis. We begin with an Inner Conversation and identify the emotions we're experiencing and what we need. Our Inner Nurturer is our source for soothing, and she validates our emotions and uses soothing words and a soothing tone to provide calm, comfort, and reassurance.

When we are new to the process of having Inner Conversations, we can easily slip back to our old habitual patterns for reducing pain. We quickly grab something to eat or drink, turn on the television, surf the web, or find some other distraction.

In a group therapy session, Lisa, a single, exacting, and hardworking thirty-six-year-old attorney, expressed the following concerns:

Lisa: I'm doing much better at stopping when I want to grab food and having an Inner Conversation. I'm talking back to my Inner Critic more often, and I'm even acting more loving toward myself. Yet I still find that many times per week, I don't stop and have an Inner Conversation, and I overeat and go numb. I'll never lose weight this way.

Julie: It's great that you're establishing a loving alliance between your Inner Nurturer and your *feeling self*. I'm wondering if these are times when you experience very intense, unpleasant emotional states and choose to comfort yourself with food and to numb out rather than stay connected?

Lisa: Yes, definitely. I can think of two times when that happened this week. One is when I made a mistake at work and I felt so angry with myself and ashamed. I headed right to the staff room and ate two pastries. The other time was after I spent time with my sister, who regularly criticizes and judges me. I went home and ate ice cream. I guess I felt angry and ashamed then as well.

Group member: I can't handle those emotions, either. But I wouldn't have stopped at two pastries!

Julie: When we feel that upset, we need to soothe and calm ourselves. It sounds like you're disconnecting from yourself during these times because you don't know *how* to soothe yourself. When you feel angry and ashamed, what does your Inner Nurturer say to your *feeling self*?

Lisa: At those times, it's like I lose contact with my Inner Nurturer. Or maybe she abandons me. I guess she's saying, "I don't know what to do for you. This sucks. Let's go have something yummy; you deserve it." And then I grab food.

Julie: We need to strengthen your Inner Nurturer's capability to soothe your *feeling self* and help her move through these unpleasant emotional states rather than indulge her with food.

"How Do I Soothe Myself?"

Most of us have had some exposure to soothing others, even if only briefly. Whom have you found to be soothing in your life? Maybe it was a grandparent, aunt, teacher, mentor, therapist, or family friend. Think about what exactly was soothing about this person. Was it her tone, eye contact, or touch? Did she use reassuring, kind words or offer hope and encouragement?

Now think about a situation in your life that's upsetting you. See if you can say something soothing to yourself using the voice and tone of this soothing person.

How does it feel to say soothing phrases to yourself? Foreign and awkward, like when you first started using the voice of your Inner Nurturer? Does your own voice feel even the slightest bit soothing? If not, why is it that you don't consider your own voice soothing? What qualities do you attribute to others who can soothe that you don't attribute to yourself? How is it that you can soothe a friend, small child, or suffering animal but not yourself?

The reality is that *you* know what *you* need to hear, more than anyone else. You are in the best position to give this to yourself. Your own voice can be just as soothing as anyone else's voice. It's all about practice. The more often you practice self-soothing, the easier it gets and the more comforting your own voice feels.

"It's Not Fair" and "I Don't Want To"

At this point, you may feel resistant to learning these skills. Many emotional eaters do not find it gratifying to hear me tell them that I can teach them to self-soothe. They missed out on getting their needs met by others

Soothing Words

Here are some examples of phrases your Inner Nurturer can say to your *feeling self* during an Inner Conversation.

"It's okay to feel these feelings; they are real and valid."
"I can understand being upset about this."
"I'm sorry you are going through this."
"I know this is a difficult time for you."
"I am here to help."
"Your needs are very important."
"I can take care of you and help you meet your needs."
"You can count on me."
"I love and care about you."
"I am here for you always."
"I am here with you, and we will get through this together."
"You are not alone."
"You are safe here with me."
"We'll get through this rough phase one step at a time."
"This too shall pass."
"We'll take baby steps together — come on, hold my hand."
"Everything will be all right."
"Sometimes scary things like this happen. I am here with you. I know you are scared. I'm right by your side."
"I know it seems like things keep getting worse. The tide will turn, and better days will be here."
"I believe in you. I know that together we can improve this situation."
"It's okay to make mistakes."
"You don't have to be perfect for me to love you."
"We'll do the best we can; that's all we can do."

who might have nurtured them, and they resent the notion of having to soothe themselves. It seems hard, just "one more thing to do." They tell me: "It's not fair — I don't want to have to do this for myself."

Your resistance is a sign that you're not yet fully on board with adult-like self-care. The emotions that are surfacing right now, like anger, sadness, resentment, rebellion, and even denial, are part of the grieving process. You may need to grieve the fact that you were not adequately soothed and comforted in childhood. You were left in unpleasant emotional states without assistance. Your needs were not met. And now you will have to learn to do this for yourself. It just does not seem fair.

Soothing Behaviors

When we are distressed, our emotions are intense and our thoughts can be obsessive, anxious, fearful, negative, and hopeless. We can't think clearly, and we're not functioning at our best. At these times our Inner Nurturer can suggest different soothing behaviors so that we can calm down and restore balance.

Soothing Behaviors

When you feel too agitated or upset to begin an Inner Conversation, try calming yourself with any of the following behaviors. Note that these are all meant to be done alone.

- Put on comfortable clothing.
- Sit in a comfortable chair or couch.
- Breathe deeply.
- Hold or hug yourself.
- Stroke your face, arms, and shoulders.
- Curl up in the fetal position.
- Hold a cuddly stuffed animal.
- Journal about your feelings.
- Take a warm bath or shower.
- Listen to comforting music.
- Listen to uplifting audio messages or affirmations.
- Sing.
- Play a musical instrument.
- Do yoga or stretching exercises.
- Walk or hike in nature.
- Garden.
- View or create artwork.
- Knit, bead, sew, or do needlepoint or woodworking.
- Do light housework or chores.
- Meditate.
- Pray or chant.

We use soothing behaviors to restore ourselves to calm, *not* to distract ourselves. Our goal is to calm down enough to begin an effective Inner Conversation. We need to take a look at the situation causing distress. We want to identify our emotions and stay with them. We need to make an action plan to meet our needs. And we will want to reframe any disempowering thoughts.

You do not want to use soothing behaviors to numb out. You already know how to do that with food, television, the Internet, sleeping, and shopping. When you tranquilize yourself, you don't learn or practice new skills. It will take consistent practice to develop self-soothing skills.

"Normally, I Would Have Binged"

After a few weeks of practicing soothing words and behaviors, Lisa shared in group the following success:

> Lisa: Last week, there was a power outage at our condo complex. The garage gate was open, and I pulled in. But it was pitch-black, and even with my headlights it was difficult to see. I thought I cleared the pole next to my parking space, but didn't, and I heard a loud crunch. I had just scraped up my one-month-old, new car!
>
> Group member: Oh my God! You must have been unbelievably upset. I would have been ready to kill myself!
>
> Lisa: I was. *And then I remembered that this is when I need to practice self-soothing.* I was so angry, and I needed to let out some energy to calm down, so I went inside and got on the treadmill. I would have never done that in the past! At the same time, I was soothing myself — telling myself it was okay to make a mistake — it's only metal and some money. I have insurance, et cetera. I also decided I wouldn't tell my mother about it, so I would avoid being criticized. Normally, I would have gone inside and called her and then binged. But I didn't do either.
>
> Group member: Good for you. That's impressive!

Lisa: What is so great is that I didn't have any desire to emotionally eat. I knew I needed to calm down and soothe myself.
And once I was calm, I realized that accidents happen and no
one was hurt. I made an action plan to call my insurance company the next morning and get the car into the repair shop. I
made a healthy dinner and even did *more* soothing behaviors.
I took a bath, relaxed for the evening, and felt very proud of
myself. I felt very grown-up.

When we're ready to learn and practice self-soothing skills, it's a sign
that we're willing to take responsibility for our lives and meet our own
needs. We're willing to get on with the business of learning skills we did
not adequately acquire in childhood. We're tired of feeling like victims,
of blaming ourselves and others for our current situations.

We've grown weary of living in a stagnant, passive coping state of
"It's not fair" and "I don't want to." We realize no one is going to come
and rescue us. We want to learn how to move through unpleasant emotional states and restore ourselves to hope, possibility, and fruitful action.
We are ready for effective solutions.

When Soothing Isn't Enough

Another group member, Jackie, a self-employed accountant with a playful
sense of humor, was regularly feeling upset and depressed about her relationship with her boyfriend, Sam. Soothing words and behaviors didn't
seem to relieve the depression, despair, and associated binges. Jackie, at
age forty-one, found that her biological clock was ticking loudly, and
while she wanted to settle down with Sam and start a family, she wondered if they were truly right for each other.

Sam had a lot of hobbies and friends and liked to spend a considerable
amount of time with the guys. Jackie felt like everything in his life took
precedence over spending time with her. She knew that her issues with
Sam were related to the painful childhood experiences she'd had with her

father, but she wasn't sure whether her expectations of Sam were reasonable or not.

Her mother and father had divorced when she was a young child. The custody plan had stated that Jackie, their only child, would spend two weekends per month with her father. She looked forward to these weekends very much. Her father, a busy film director, was, however, rarely able to spend two full weekends with her. He often pawned her off on his sister or mother or other family members. When he was with her, he was distracted by work and other personal matters.

Jackie thought she had finished grieving her childhood experiences of neglect and invisibility in therapy years earlier. But she realized that even though she had spent plenty of time crying, she had spent more time numbing herself with food and that her Inner Nurturer was nonexistent. She feared that her neediness was a turnoff to Sam and pushed him away. She felt powerless to change their situation and hopeless about their future.

She was unconsciously looking for Sam to "make it all better."

Grieving Is the Healing Self-Care Skill

In our fast-paced Western culture, discussion about our painful inner experiences is discouraged. Talking about our pain is considered a sign of weakness and evidence that we're not getting on with our lives. Needless to say, we don't have too high an opinion of grieving, either. We don't like to grieve — it's a painful process and there often is no immediate end in sight. We expect the grieving process to be brief and done in private. We steer clear of people who are grieving. Other people's grief brings up our own unhealed wounds and unmourned losses.

We know we are supposed to grieve severe losses such as the death of a loved one or a painful divorce. But what about the losses we experience because of a neglect-filled, traumatic childhood? What about the time and opportunities lost during the years we are dysfunctional and numbing ourselves with food? If we are to acquire good emotional health, these losses must be mourned as well.

If we expand our perspective and look beyond the immediate discomfort of grieving, we will see that it is a process of adaptation and growth, one not to be discounted or avoided.

Grieving is a transformative process, one that leads to renewal, hope, and the possibility for creative change. It requires willingness, patience, and courage as we move through the many emotions and stages of grieving. It demands a leap of faith — faith that if we go through this dark tunnel, there will be some relief and something better on the other side. That at some point the grief will lessen and we will begin to feel a sense of renewal and will gain an expanded perspective.

Old Pain

Most of us don't spend much time thinking about our losses, disappointments, or painful childhood experiences. We are reminded of our losses when something in our environment triggers thoughts of them. We see a happy couple and think, "I was once part of a happy couple, until Joe cheated on me." We witness a mother yelling at her child in the supermarket and for a brief moment remember what it felt like to be a child with a screaming mother. We witness a chubby child interacting with his friends on the playground and immediately remember the shame and criticism we experienced as an overweight kid. And then the cell phone rings and our thoughts shift to more pressing matters.

So why should we dredge up all those painful memories? Without your realizing it, those painful experiences you've pushed out of your awareness are fueling your emotional eating, highly reactive emotional states, low motivation, anxiety, depression, and relationship difficulties. I realize this may seem odd, because you truly believe your overeating is due to a lack of willpower and difficulty coping with current problems or situations. But in truth, your current pain is often just the tip of a big iceberg of pain buried deep within, what I call "old pain."

Our bodies and brains are like computers in the sense that they have a seemingly endless capability to store memories, both pleasant and unpleasant. But unlike computers, they have no delete button we can use to trash unwanted memory files. We have to resort to maladaptive coping patterns and defense mechanisms to keep our old pain from rearing up. And while these behaviors and ego defenses protect us by blocking out old pain, they require energy and can put a damper on our vitality and motivation.

There is a better way. While we may not be able to get rid of old, painful memories, we can release the emotional pain stored with them, so that when they do surface they no longer carry a strong negative charge. Just as a battery still exists after it has used up its power, these old memories will still exist but will have no power to unbalance us and fuel emotional eating.

Trauma and Highly Reactive Emotional States

Researchers have demonstrated that even mild levels of routine criticism, blame, shame, and neglect can be experienced as traumatizing and can affect brain development. The combination of chronic stress, trauma, and restricted emotional expression that we experience in dysfunctional families can produce long-lasting and perhaps permanent changes in brain neuron excitability. As we continue to encounter painful experiences in childhood, neuronal pathways become enlarged or deeply grooved and new pathways may be carved out. The result is that people exposed to trauma often have difficulty regulating emotional arousal and are more prone to anxiety and depression. Their brains seem to be primed to overreact to situations that feel similar to the original painful experiences.

As children, we tend to consider these painful experiences normal because we don't know anything different. But they are not normal or healthy for our development and can have long-lasting effects on our emotional well-being.

Trauma can be defined as any experience that is startling or damaging and that has a lasting effect on mental health. The traumas you might have experienced in childhood are listed in table 3, "Core Traumas."

Painful childhood experiences may have been the result of intentional behaviors on the part of our caregivers, such as shaming, attacking, or rejecting us. They may also have been caused by unintentional behaviors outside our caregivers' control. The abandonment we experience from the illness or death of a caregiver is traumatic but unintentional. Caregivers who are fragmenting or falling apart under pressure may unintentionally ignore our needs or overload us with an inappropriate level of adult responsibilities. Some of our painful experiences, like neglect, betrayal, and blame, may have occurred repeatedly, whereas others, like sexual abuse, may have occurred once or twice and never again.

When you read the description of a core trauma, all aspects of the description may not fit your particular case. For example, if you underwent the core trauma "deprivation or neglect," you may have experienced a lack of soothing, recognition, and validation, but limits were strictly enforced and not lacking. If any of the traumas listed in table 3 occurred frequently during your developing years, or they occurred infrequently but were unsettling, I would consider them core traumas. They have adversely affected your mental health.

If you began to use food for emotional comfort early in life, you have most likely experienced some trauma in your childhood. Many emotional eaters tell me they experienced quite a few of the traumas listed in table 3. Keep in mind that your reaction to trauma is unique. It is influenced by many factors, including severity and frequency, your genetic constitution or sturdiness, and any counterbalancing positive influences in the environment.

When Trauma *Feels Like a Strong Word*

Perhaps *trauma* is a word you have associated only with *severe* physical, emotional, or sexual abuse. It never occurred to you to apply the word to the rage, criticism, rejection, scapegoating, emotional unavailability, or low level of neglect you experienced as a child. You never thought being assigned excessive responsibility for the care of elders or siblings was *traumatic*. Sure your father criticized you regularly and was impatient with you, but it was because *you* were not a good student or *you* had a learning disability or *he* was "just under a lot of pressure." Yes, your mother yelled and screamed throughout your childhood, but did that really constitute *trauma*?

Emotional eating and mood disturbances such as anxiety and depression point to the fact that your childhood experiences *were* mildly to severely traumatizing and *did* derail your development. In order to resolve your overeating, you must accept the fact that your childhood experiences did have an impact on your mental health. Your trust in others has been betrayed and you have learned not to trust your own emotional signals. Parts of your emotional development have been frozen in time because of this unresolved pain.

It's not that we want to view ourselves as perpetual victims and forever blame our wounded caregivers. Or wear our old pain as a badge of honor and retell our story over and over as a self-indulgent means of getting attention. We want to heal, and we cannot heal if we do not acknowledge that something very wrong and painful happened to us. We seek recovery; that is, we seek to recover our vibrant, creative, authentic self that got buried under layers of emotional pain.

Acknowledging that trauma occurred in your childhood may feel shameful. It means admitting you and your caregivers are flawed. Do you feel that acknowledging your experiences as trauma means that your childhood was not as good as you would like to remember it or that your caregivers were not as loving as you would like to believe? Maybe you feel disloyal to the people who raised you. They may have passed on and so are not here to defend themselves. Sometimes just the act of acknowledging our resistance to the word *trauma* is enough to release it.

If the word *trauma* still feels like it doesn't quite fit your particular experiences, try substituting the term *core issues* or *core wounds*.

Table 3

Core Traumas

ABANDONMENT	Emotional or physical withdrawal, unavailability, or desertion. This can be the result of having a workaholic or substance-abusing caregiver or of the caregiver's temporary or permanent absence due to illness, death, or desertion.
ATTACK	Verbal or physical anger, aggression, assault, or violence; harsh criticism.
BETRAYAL	Result of caregivers' chronic unfaithfulness in guarding or maintaining trust; broken confidences, unpredictability, deception, or broken or empty promises.
BLAME	Being held responsible for the feelings, actions, faults, or errors of others.
DECEPTION	Being intentionally misled regarding facts, feelings, needs, and behaviors.
DEPRIVATION OR NEGLECT	Result of caregivers' lack of attention to, and lack of care for, emotional or physical needs; lack of recognition and validation; lack of empathy, soothing, kindness, and warmth; poor emotional attunement; a lack of emotional availability, wise guidance, patience, good listening, and interest; unjust punishments; or a lack of limits.
DOMINATION	Being controlled; encouragement of dependency and submissiveness, and punishment for autonomous, independent behavior.
ENGULFMENT	Exposure to continual invasion of emotional or physical boundaries; smothering.
EXPLOITATION	Being used to serve others' purposes, either positively (for example, as a prideful extension) or negatively (for example, being made to do excessive and age-inappropriate chores).
FRAGMENTATION	Exposure to caregivers who are overwhelmed and unstable, anxious, depressed, falling apart, delusional, or dissociative.

(continued)

Table 3	
Core Traumas (continued)	
PARENTIFICATION	Being expected to be a "little grown-up" and inappropriately care for others (parents, siblings, or other family members).
REJECTION	Being dismissed, ignored, treated as useless, unsatisfactory, inadequate, invisible, unwanted, or worthless; being scapegoated or cast out.
SHAME	Humiliation as a result of being criticized regularly, especially in front of others.
VIOLATION	Exposure to personal boundary transgressions — for example, violence or sexual abuse.

Highly Reactive Emotional States

Stressful situations and even seemingly ordinary interactions can trigger intense emotional states for those who have experienced trauma. These are times when deep emotional wounds are activated and we experience old, familiar, unpleasant emotions like anxiety, rage, depression, and jealousy. Think about times when someone said something to you, or did something, and you felt an intense reaction that did not subside or fade quickly. You've probably experienced these emotions many times in the past and have been stuck in them for hours, days, or longer.

When we experience these intense feelings, our thoughts can be obsessive as we revisit and reanalyze the triggering event. Our behavior is often compulsive; we may have a strong impulse to lash out at another or withdraw and isolate ourselves. We may act out the pain on ourselves with self-destructive behaviors such as hitting or cutting. We may become clingy and compliant as we try to merge with the hurtful other and restore emotional balance. This is prime time for soothing and numbing activities like emotional eating.

Highly Reactive Emotional States

During a highly reactive emotional state, you may feel any of the following:

Agitation	Frustration	Obligation
Anxiety	Guilt	Overwhelmed
Confusion	Helplessness	Powerlessness
Depression	Hopelessness	Rage
Disappointment	Hostility	Resentment
Disgust	Hurt	Responsibility
Emptiness	Insecurity	Sadness
Entitlement	Invisibility	Shame
Envy	Jealousy	Shock
Fear	Loneliness	Unworthiness
Fragmentation	Neediness	Vulnerability

Triggers for Highly Reactive Emotional States

+ Losses and disappointments
+ Confrontations or arguments
+ Shame, criticism, judgment, or attack
+ Rejection, dismissal, or scapegoating
+ Not being listened to or understood
+ Abandonment or exclusion
+ Deprivation
+ Too much responsibility or stress
+ Seeing yourself in a mirror or photograph
+ Loss of control
+ Handling something poorly
+ Breakups
+ Betrayals of trust
+ Milestone events: births, deaths, graduations, weddings, baby showers, and so on

My Personal Experience with Grieving

I learned firsthand about the healing power of grieving and the necessity of working through painful childhood experiences when I began weekly psychotherapy in my twenties. It was the best decision and investment I ever made. To the outside world, it might have appeared that I had it all together. I had a master's degree in business administration from the University of California, Los Angeles, and was working for a large, prestigious accounting firm. I had a promising career ahead and a loving boyfriend. On the inside, however, I was a wreck. I was suffering from chronic bouts of anxiety and depression. I had low self-esteem and a poor body image. I was perfectionistic and highly critical of myself. I rarely felt I did a good enough job at anything. I medicated myself nightly with food.

My therapist gently and lovingly encouraged me to "revisit and grieve" the traumatic events of my childhood. At times I resisted, wondering how discussing my mother's bipolar illness and rage fests or my father's emotional unavailability would help me stop overeating or feel less anxious and depressed *now*. After all, those events were in the past. She reassured me that talking about my painful childhood experiences and actually reexperiencing the original repressed feelings would help lift some of the depression and reduce the need to numb myself. Even though I wanted more immediate relief, I put my trust in her because nothing I was doing was working.

As I revisited the losses, disappointments, traumatic events, and painful experiences of my childhood, my therapist empathically listened and validated my pain. It seemed as if, for the first time in my life, I was experiencing mirroring, empathy, and consistent kindness.

The floodgates opened and I began to grieve regularly, often daily, in and out of therapy. I stuck with the process, as painful as it was, because I was experiencing many benefits. I felt emotionally lighter — less anxious and less depressed. I felt heard, seen, validated, and not so alone in my pain. I was learning to be less critical of myself and more compassionate as I began to internalize my therapist's kind, nurturing voice. My resistance, rigidity, and defensiveness were softening. I was feeling more hopeful, and all of this translated into a reduction in my emotional eating.

Resolving Old Pain

My intention here is to provide you with an understanding of the skills required to process losses, disappointments, highly reactive emotional states, and the old, painful childhood experiences underneath them. Revisiting and grieving these experiences can be painful work. While I have provided a three-step "Retreat, Revisit, and Grieve" process to practice, I believe it is best for everyone beginning the process of working through childhood trauma to work with an experienced psychotherapist. These are difficult skills to learn and practice on your own.

An experienced professional can lovingly guide you through your natural resistance to accessing old memories and experiencing unpleasant emotions. She can provide a safe space to allow repressed memories to surface. She can validate your emotions and model the kind, soothing, supportive, and nonjudgmental voice of the Inner Nurturer. She can help you strengthen your self-soothing skills. She can help you build up internal and external resources. She can contain and help you regulate intense emotions and set an appropriate pace for working through your pain. And she can determine whether additional therapeutic modalities for working through trauma — such as eye-movement desensitization and reprocessing, and emotional freedom techniques that utilize tapping on energy points — or other body-oriented therapies might be beneficial.

Your motivation to go through this process will be higher with an experienced guide, and you can process and resolve old pain in a shorter amount of time.

We All Want a Quick Fix

There are no quick fixes for resolving the losses and old pain left over from a dysfunctional childhood. If you are overeating or bingeing regularly, having difficulty managing your weight, feeling challenged by anxiety or depression, and chronically overreacting to situations in your life, you are living with the aftereffects of unmourned loss and trauma.

Depending on the severity and frequency of the trauma(s) you have experienced and its impact on you, you may be processing your old pain for many years to come. Keep in mind that it is not something you will have to do every day or even every week. It's something you will *choose* to do when you feel like disconnecting from yourself and numbing or lashing out. These are the times when the iceberg is surfacing and you have to go inside and melt more of it down.

The more you practice these processing skills, the quicker you will be able to discharge old pain and rebalance yourself. Just as you will continue to exercise and eat healthy food the rest of your life, you will use your "retreat, revisit, and grieve" skills forever.

At times you have to push yourself to exercise and prepare healthy food. In the same way, you will have to push yourself some of the time to clear out your old pain. Remind yourself of all the benefits you receive from doing this work and how great you feel afterward.

Even though I no longer eat emotionally, I still experience the aftereffects of a childhood filled with loss and trauma. When I feel highly reactive or mildly depressed, I actually look forward to sitting down with my journal and releasing the pain. I am confident I will feel better afterward and gain a new perspective on the situation and my life.

If you choose to try these exercises on your own, it's a good idea to have a trusted, supportive friend present or available afterward for sharing. Take it slow during this process; there is no rush. It took years to build up this old pain, and it will take time to resolve it. If you feel overwhelmed, stop the exercises immediately.

CAUTION: Do not try these exercises on your own if any of the following apply. It will be best, in that case, to access and process your emotions with the help of, and in the presence of, a professional psychotherapist.

- When experiencing intense emotions, you feel like you are going to break down or fall apart, or you have felt this sense of falling apart before and it took you days or weeks to recover.

- You have been diagnosed with any mental illness, including post–traumatic stress disorder.
- You have been hospitalized in the past with a mental illness.
- There is mental illness in your family.
- You have been the victim of severe physical, sexual, or emotional abuse or trauma.

Practicing the Three-Step "Retreat, Revisit, and Grieve" Process

You can use this three-step process whenever any of the following apply:

- You have a strong desire to eat and you're not hungry.
- You are hungry and want to binge or choose unhealthy comfort food.
- You want to eat beyond fullness.
- You want to disconnect from yourself and numb out with activities like watching television, surfing the Internet, playing video games, shopping, creating drama, having sex, gambling, or overworking.
- You are experiencing unpleasant emotions.
- You are in a highly reactive emotional state.

These are the times your mind, body, and spirit are signaling you that the iceberg is surfacing.

Preparing a Safe Space

Create a safe womb-like space at home where you can practice your "retreat, revisit, and grieve" skills. This space might include a comfortable chair, a couch, a stack of pillows, a warm blanket, favorite stuffed animals, pictures of yourself as a child, candles, and anything else you find soothing. As you gain experience in processing painful childhood experiences, you'll be able to practice these skills anywhere. I've done this work on planes and trains, in airport and restaurant bathrooms, in hotels, in my car — you name it.

Keep a special "old pain" journal in your safe space. If you fear someone will read your journal, you may want to find a safe hiding place or, if necessary, tear up your writings as you go. The point here is not to memorialize your pain but rather to get the emotions out of your body. Instruct others not to disturb you when you are in this space.

Preparing Yourself

You'll need to set aside thirty to sixty minutes of undisturbed time to practice these skills. Sit quietly and allow yourself to feel the comfort and safety of this special place. Take a few moments to relax your body; stretch your head from side to side and then tense and release all the muscle groups from your shoulders to your feet. Focus on your breathing: breathe in calm, breathe out tension.

Retreat, Revisit, and Grieve

STEP 1. **RETREAT** to a safe space and identify the situation or inner conflict causing distress. Identify the emotions you are experiencing and how they feel in your body.

STEP 2. Scan your memory bank as far back as possible for times when you felt this same feeling state. Any memory will do. **REVISIT** and replay the situation(s) in your mind, as if you're watching a video of it, remembering it as best you can and reexperiencing the associated emotions. Don't worry about accuracy.

STEP 3. **GRIEVE** the story with all its details.

Step 1. Retreat to a safe space and identify the situation or inner conflict causing distress. Identify the emotions you are experiencing and how they feel in your body.

When you're in a situation that causes you distress, especially if it causes a highly reactive emotional state, you need to remove yourself from the situation. It's best not to engage others when you're in an agitated state, even though the urge to react may be strong. There is a high probability that you will distort what you hear and will say things you'll later regret. Change the subject or ask to revisit the discussion at a later date, and politely excuse yourself. Remove yourself from food, distracting activities, and other people. If you can get yourself to a safe, quiet place where you can be alone and explore your emotions and the possible old pain being triggered, proceed to step 2.

If you don't have the time to process right now, then substitute a quick, soothing Inner Conversation. Life is busy and hectic, and generally we don't have thirty to sixty minutes available on the spot for processing old pain. At such times we need to contain our pain, self-soothe, and temporarily restore balance. Make time later that day or the next to go back to the situation causing distress and proceed to step 2, even if you feel as if you're over the issue. Otherwise it may cause unconscious emotional eating in the days ahead.

Write in your journal what you believe is causing distress. If it feels like a jumble of many issues, list anything and everything. List both external stressors (the fight with your best friend) and internal stressors (the dissatisfaction with your body). Pick one issue to focus on that feels most significant.

See self-care skill #1, in chapter 2, for a review of identifying and experiencing emotions. As you name each emotion, see if you can locate these emotions in your body. Stay with them.

If you have the time and space to proceed to step 2, in the next section, but find that you are too agitated or overwhelmed to begin, engage in a nonfood, noncompulsive soothing behavior, such as listening to music or doing some deep breathing, to calm yourself enough to begin the work.

EXAMPLE

On the way to her office, Jackie has a big argument with her boyfriend, Sam. When she arrives at work, her assistant reminds her of an important client meeting in twenty minutes, and all Jackie can think of is getting two brownies and a latte from the coffee shop on the first floor. Instead, she closes the door to her office and decides to have a quick soothing Inner Conversation.

Later that evening, Jackie pulls out her journal and writes about the argument with Sam regarding plans for the upcoming weekend. He routinely makes plans without consulting her and has already committed to plans for the weekend. She had hoped for some quality alone-time together.

Jackie writes that she is *feeling* angry, hurt, agitated, anxious, sad, lonely, hopeless, powerless, and disappointed. She feels the anger and powerlessness as tension throughout her whole body. The sadness, loneliness, hurt, hopelessness, and disappointment present as an achy feeling in her upper body. She also notices that the anxiety and agitation feel like restlessness and a difficulty sitting still and concentrating.

Step 2. Scan your memory bank as far back as possible for times when you felt this same feeling state. Any memory will do. Revisit and replay the situation(s) in your mind, as if you're watching a video of it, remembering it as best you can and reexperiencing the associated emotions. Don't worry about accuracy.

Go back as far as you can, even to infancy if you have memories of that. If you can't access any childhood memories, try to access an early-adulthood memory. Ask yourself the following questions to help access memories:

"Does this situation or this person's reaction or behavior remind me of a painful experience I had when I was younger?"

"Does this person remind me of anyone from the past — Mom, Dad, Grandma, Grandpa, or an aunt, uncle, sister, brother, neighbor, family friend, teacher, rabbi, priest, or someone else?"

"Do I remember a time long ago when I felt these same intense feelings?"

"Is this situation or conflict touching off, or reminding me of, any
   painful losses?"

The goal here is to access and reexperience the original repressed
emotions resulting from painful childhood experiences. The accuracy
of the details is not important — what you think you remember is good
enough. Stay with these emotions as they surface. Locate them in your
body. You are beginning the grieving process now. You may want to hold
yourself or a stuffed animal as you reexperience this pain.

To return to my example: Jackie sits back and closes her eyes as she
feels these emotions. She realizes that this situation with Sam reminds
her of the numerous occasions she looked forward to spending time with
her father, only to be disappointed when he canceled their plans at the
last minute. Jackie replays in her mind one time in particular, her eighth
birthday, when he promised to take her and her best girlfriend up to a
local mountain resort for a weekend of ski lessons and fun in the snow. He
was to pick them up Friday night, and they would head to the mountains
Saturday morning. She and her girlfriend had their bags packed and were
ready to go Friday night. Her father called Friday night to say that something had come up and he would still try to make it Saturday morning, but
not to count on it. He said he would make it up to her if he couldn't go.
Jackie had heard unfulfilled promises like these many times.

That night, she was inconsolable. She had looked forward to this trip
for months, in spite of her mother's warnings not to get her hopes up. She
felt unimportant and invisible to her father. It was clear that everything
else in his life was more important than her. She felt depressed and hopeless about ever feeling loved and cherished by him.

Her father never called the next morning, and even though Jackie's
mother tried her best to make the day special, Jackie felt disappointed and
downhearted all day.

Step 3. Grieve the story with all its details.

Journal freely, writing in detail about the situation, the painful memories, your emotions, longings, unmet needs, losses, and disappointments.

You can cry, rage, scream, *and* write, or allow yourself to feel your feelings first and then write. Write down anything that comes to mind, without censorship. This may include expletives and angry, critical comments. Don't skip the writing part. You will find that you stay with your emotions and the grieving process more fully when you journal.

Grief is a mixture of many emotions. You may experience conflicting emotions: you may feel hatred and anger toward the person in your memory *and* guilt for feeling this way. Feel free to make noise as you grieve — weep, scream, rant, hit a pillow, and stomp. *This is your old pain.* There is nothing to *do* with it except to *be* with it. You are melting the iceberg of old pain each time you grieve. Yes, I know, it's uncomfortable. It will get easier.

By reexperiencing these repressed emotions and writing about the memories, you are connecting to your *feeling self* in an intimate way. You are confirming that these experiences did in fact happen. You are listening to and honoring your old pain. You may also choose to share these painful memories with a close friend or a therapist.

As Jackie revisits and replays this memory, she is surprised at how strong the pain still feels. It's a mixture of anger and deep sadness. First she feels the anger, intensely, in her neck and shoulders. Then comes the sadness in her chest and she begins to cry. She cries for the young child she was — the sweet little girl who just wanted to be close to her father. She grieves for the little girl who wanted to feel important, to be called Daddy's girl. Many similar memories come to the surface now, and Jackie cries and writes about these as well.

She reflects on her adolescent years spent looking for love in all the wrong places. She feels shame about the years of promiscuity and her attraction to emotionally unavailable men. She feels sad about her lack of trust in men and the fact that she still seems to be attracting the same type of man. She feels sad about how needy, clingy, and demanding she is with Sam.

She thinks about her mother, and she grieves for her mother's sadness and loneliness as well. Her mother never remarried, and Jackie has always felt her mother's pain and emptiness. She wishes she could take away her mother's pain.

Jackie is grieving the core traumas of abandonment, betrayal, rejection, deprivation/neglect, and shame.

After the Grieving

Sometime after a grieving session, you may want to continue with the following four optional steps:

Step 4. Access your Inner Nurturer for soothing and comforting words.

Even though the grieving process offers release and relief, we can feel spent afterward, just as we do after a good workout. Close out this session by reinforcing the alliance between your *feeling self* and your Inner Nurturer. Write in your journal a few reassuring phrases such as:

"I love you, _____."
"I am here with you always."
"You are safe here with me."
"I can and will take care of you."
"You can rely on me."
"We're going to be okay."

If time permits, follow up this session with soothing behaviors like listening to music, spending time with animals, reading inspirational words, gardening, or taking an easy stroll in an inspiring place. Give yourself a pat on the back for work well done.

As Jackie completes the grieving session in my example, she writes the following phrases in her journal:

"I love you, little Jackie."
"I'm sorry that you had to feel so rejected by Dad."
"Your needs *are* important, and I will make sure they are met."

"You don't have to look to Sam to meet all your needs; I am here for you."

Step 5. Make an action plan to address any unmet needs that were highlighted during the grieving session.

See self-care skill #1, in chapter 2, for a review of meeting your needs. An action plan might even include grieving more regularly.

Jackie realizes that, like her mother, she doesn't take enough time for herself. In addition, she recognizes that she gets lazy about making plans with her friends. As a result, she sets an intention to spend quality time alone or with friends every weekend. She wants to see what effect this will have on her relationship with Sam.

Step 6. Catch and reframe any self-defeating thoughts that surfaced during the grieving session.

See self-care skill #2, in chapter 3, for a review of reframing thoughts. Jackie notices that she has written the following self-defeating thought:

"No one will ever truly love me; I'm just a needy bottomless pit."

This is a core belief she adopted long ago in reaction to her father's rejection and criticism of her needs. She writes down a few energizing reframes to practice whenever this thought pops up:

"I'm not a bottomless pit — a tiny bit of the *right* kind of love fills me up immediately."
"It's perfectly okay to ask others to meet some of my needs."
"I am capable of meeting many of my needs myself."
"I am lovable as is."

Step 7. Write down any new awareness or lesson that came out of this grieving session.

Do you see yourself or your past in a new way? Do you see another person differently? Can you see your current situation in a new light?

Do you see any lessons or additional meaning in these experiences?

After the grieving session, Jackie feels a renewed sense of hope regarding her relationship with Sam. She realizes that she hasn't been taking the best care of herself and that this put pressure on their relationship. Sam was initially attracted to Jackie's independence because his own mother is very needy and engulfing. In some ways, she has become like his mother. It makes sense that he has been pulling away from her.

She reminds herself that it's okay to have expectations about spending time with Sam. She also reminds herself that *he isn't her father*, and that he used to be more emotionally and physically available. She believes that as she spends more quality time off on her own, Sam will want to spend more quality time with her.

Active Grieving

When our lives have been filled with disappointments, losses, and an inordinate amount of pain and suffering, we need to set aside time regularly to "melt the iceberg." Even if our lives have not been filled with pain and suffering, we can stay in tip-top emotional shape by setting aside time to grieve the necessary losses associated with growth and maturity. We may need time to grieve lost opportunities, an empty nest, and getting older and losing our fertility and youthful beauty.

In the months and years that follow loss, "active grieving," as I call it — purposely revisiting the loss and continuing to grieve — affords us further opportunity to assimilate the loss and grow from it. This way, we can stay flexible, positive, and hopeful. We may even choose to rewrite our story from a new, expanded perspective. When we cannot make meaning out of loss, we risk becoming bitter, resentful, and hopeless.

Our desire to emotionally eat, numb out, or act out is the signal that some pain, old or new, needs releasing. As you gain experience with this process, you will notice that it brings rapid relief as well as insight and renewal.

After (or even during) a "retreat, revisit, and grieve" session, it can be very helpful to use a grief letter to express your feelings. Always try to feel the feelings as you write them. You don't need to send the letter to anyone — it's a tool to help you process your pain.

Grief Letter

Dear _____ [address it to yourself or another person]:

This letter is regarding the following situation:

At the time, I felt:

At the time, I needed:

Today, I'm still feeling:

I can/cannot forgive:

I choose to accept:

Signed:

With This Very Important Skill Set under Your Belt...

When you practice self-soothing regularly, you release the internal stress that builds up from everyday life, and you feel emotionally lighter. Being willing to visit the "dark nights of your soul" allows you to periodically melt that iceberg of old pain you've been carrying around with you for a very long time, perhaps in the form of body fat or mood challenges.

Now that you've established a loving alliance between your Inner Nurturer and your *feeling self*, your internal world should be feeling more like the sanctuary it was meant to be. It's time to move on and strengthen your Inner Nurturer's capacity to set limits.

CHAPTER FIVE

Skill #4. Create a State of Enough-ness, Then Set Nurturing Limits

For many emotional eaters, the concept of limits is equated with deprivation. We live our lives as if there were never enough. We eat more food because there isn't enough love, attention, and care. We eat more because there isn't enough time, pleasure, joy, friendship, purpose, passion, success, sex, money, downtime, and ease. We often experience a letdown when eating time is over. The prospect of getting back to work, home, or kids doesn't feel nourishing. We overeat to fill up before we feel empty again.

We know that eating more food will not rid us of the experience of scarcity and bring about abundance. We eat because we don't know how to truly nourish ourselves and meet our needs. Perhaps we've lost hope that our needs can be met. We've never mastered the balancing act of nurturing ourselves *and* setting limits.

At times our limits seem to be nonexistent, like when we binge for days on end or shop ourselves into major credit card debt. Other times, our limits are harsh as we begin another overly restrictive diet or an exercise regimen way too intense for our out-of-shape body, with the belief that *this* time we will stick to it. We experience our inability to stick to limits as failure, further evidence of our laziness and lack of willpower or discipline.

In order to be successful at setting effective, nurturing limits with ourselves, we need to first reduce our experience of lack and limitation. In this chapter, I'll show you *how* to establish a state of enough-ness and then set nurturing limits on your own behavior and that of others.

Before Limits, There Was Enough-ness

When, as children, we feel "full" from the love and nurturance our care-givers provide, we grow up with a sense of there being enough — enough love, care, attention, safety, warmth, fun, excitement, opportunity, and hope. We venture out into the world with a deep-seated sense of enough-ness, trusting that our needs can and will be met.

Our caregivers must consistently strike a balance between providing us with enough of what we need *and* setting appropriate limits — limits to protect us from dangers we cannot yet comprehend, including our own impulses. "That's enough" is a phrase we learn to get used to. "That's enough candy and treats." "That's enough television." "That's enough play time with friends." If our caregivers adequately accomplish the task of providing us with just the right amount of nourishment while setting effective limits, we will experience limits as a form of nurturance and pro-tection, even though we rebel against them. We will learn to trust the wisdom of our caregivers and, without realizing it, begin to internalize a nurturing, limit-setting voice of our own.

When we have not had sufficient nurturance in our developing years, an exaggerated craving for nurturance persists into our adulthood. It feels like an empty space that can't be filled. It shows up in our excesses as well as in our bouts of apathy and boredom.

And whether our caregivers were lax, indulgent, or harsh or they deprived us of what we needed, we have difficulty setting effective limits because these always feel too restrictive. We have not developed a kind, firm limit-setting voice of our own.

Our difficulty with setting and enforcing limits on our own behav-ior is a signal that we are not experiencing enough of the right kind of fulfillment in our lives. We are settling for second best: *feeling full* and pleasured by food rather than being *fulfilled* by our lives. Our *feeling self* doesn't care one iota about limits, weight gain, or health problems. She wants pleasure, NOW!

We begin to establish a state of enough-ness by identifying what's missing in our lives. Stop for a moment and make a list in your journal of what is lacking in your life or what there isn't enough of. Include things like significant relationships, downtime, joy, meaningful work, hobbies, and the like.

"How Could There Ever Be Enough?"

When I first began working with Barbara, she was newly divorced. She had been married to a very successful entertainment industry executive for twenty-five years. They had no children, and Barbara had not worked outside the home during their marriage. She lamented that "Jack was rigid and controlling; and even though I wasn't fulfilled in the marriage, I feel lost without him. I never realized how dependent I was on him."

Shy and reserved at age fifty-two, with few friends and little family, she found herself lacking the skills to go out in the world and create a new life for herself. Depressed and anxious, she engaged in nightly binges that became her main source of soothing, comfort, and pleasure. Feeling empty inside, she wondered how she would ever feel there was enough love and care in her life.

Barbara's wish list looked like this:

What is lacking in my life, or what isn't there enough of?

1. A kind, loving partner
2. Quality friendships
3. Good listening
4. Affection
5. Fun
6. Purpose or meaning

Even though you may not be able to easily or immediately fulfill your desired wish list, it's important to write it down. Getting clear on what's missing is an important first step in taking the best care of yourself and manifesting your desires. One thing is clear — eating *more* food will not help to bring the items on your list into your life.

The next two steps involve both creativity and commitment. First, identify at least one nonfood way to bring more of each item into your life. List only those commitments you can truly say yes to. If an item on your list involves another person or people, see if there is a way you could give yourself what's missing until more people show up in your life. Keep in mind that good self-care is very attractive to others. Second, set an intention and time frame for following through with the commitments on your list.

Here is Barbara's expanded list:

1. A kind, loving partner: Well, I guess I need to work on being kind and loving to myself as a start. I tend to be pretty hard on myself. I need to get back to practicing my Inner Conversations and catching and reframing my critical thoughts. I'll do this weekly for the next month, and then maybe I'll feel ready to sign up for a three-month trial on a dating site.

2. Quality friendships: While I don't feel up to going out and making new friends at this time, I think I could be a better friend to the few friends I have by calling them more often just to say hello.

3. Good listening: My therapist is the only one I get this from right now. When I journal regularly, I feel like I listen better to myself. I'll start with that and commit to journaling at least a few times each week.

4. Affection: I've been thinking about adopting a cat — maybe it's time to do that. I'll check out pet adoptions within the next month.

5. Fun: I love to see movies and haven't gone in a long time. I'll take in a movie this weekend, either with a friend or by myself.

6. Purpose or meaning: I could address this and the cat-adoption issue at the same time — I'll check into volunteering with a local cat-rescue group.

The final step to creating a state of enough-ness is to monitor your progress. A busy life can easily get in the way of your best intentions. Be specific about how and when you will complete the activities on your list. Set a reminder in your calendar to check up on yourself to see if you've followed through on your stated goals. If you've missed the mark, be gentle with yourself *and* set another date for completion or, if necessary, modify your goal.

Creating a State of Enough-ness

+ Make a detailed listing of what there isn't enough of in your life.
+ Identify at least one nonfood way to bring more of each item on your list into your life. Be creative.
+ Set an intention and a time frame for following through with the activities you've listed.
+ Monitor your progress.

Once your daily and weekly life includes more enjoyable, nourishing experiences, you're ready to practice some gentle limit-setting.

Strengthening the Voice of the Inner Limit-Setter

We begin the process of *setting nurturing limits* with ourselves by practicing Limit-Setting Inner Conversations. It may seem challenging to set limits with your *feeling self* when she is demanding and impulsive. In the beginning she may win out more often than you would like.

Your current attempts at limit setting may sound like this:

Feeling Self: "Let's go down the candy aisle and get some chocolate."

Inner Nurturer (as Inner Limit-Setter): "Better not; we already ate too much junk this weekend. Let's just go home, and we'll have some fruit for dessert."

Feeling Self: "No, I want chocolate. Can't we just have a little candy tonight?"

Inner Nurturer (as Inner Indulger): "Okay, we deserve a treat. Then we'll start clean tomorrow."

Feeling Self: "Wow, I love the way these shoes look. I want them."

Inner Nurturer (as Inner Limit-Setter): "They are way too expensive, and we need to stick to the budget and not spend any more money."

Feeling Self: "But it's hard to find shoes that fit, that I like, in this color. I want them! I need them!"

Inner Nurturer (as Inner Indulger): "All right. What's a little more debt on the credit card? And we do have tax-return money coming."

You'll need to become conscious of these conversations and slowly begin to strengthen the limit-setting capability of your Inner Nurturer. Your Inner Nurturer must do her job as an Inner Limit-Setter and set a nurturing limit. When your *feeling self* resists, your Inner Nurturer steps in and finds out what she is truly longing for or what she feels there is not enough of. Your Inner Nurturer also reassures your *feeling self* that her needs can be met.

Your new, effective Limit-Setting Inner Conversations will sound like this:

Feeling Self: "Let's go down the candy aisle and get some chocolate."

Inner Nurturer (as Inner Limit-Setter): "Better not; we already ate too much junk this weekend. Let's just go home, and we'll have some fruit for dessert."

Feeling Self: "No, I want chocolate. Can't we just have a little candy tonight?"

Inner Nurturer: "I know you're not hungry, so tell me what you're feeling; what are you truly longing for right now, other than candy?"

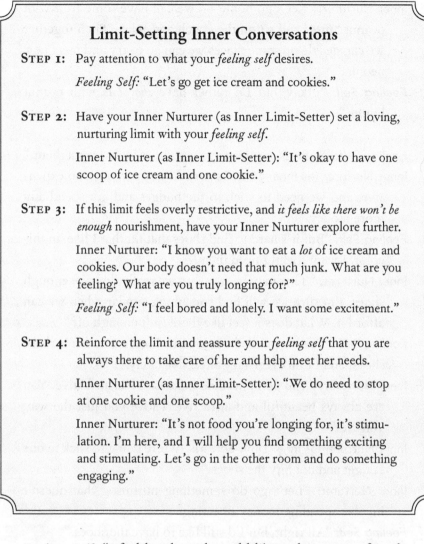

Limit-Setting Inner Conversations

STEP 1: Pay attention to what your *feeling self* desires.

Feeling Self: "Let's go get ice cream and cookies."

STEP 2: Have your Inner Nurturer (as Inner Limit-Setter) set a loving, nurturing limit with your *feeling self*.

Inner Nurturer (as Inner Limit-Setter): "It's okay to have one scoop of ice cream and one cookie."

STEP 3: If this limit feels overly restrictive, and *it feels like there won't be enough* nourishment, have your Inner Nurturer explore further.

Inner Nurturer: "I know you want to eat a *lot* of ice cream and cookies. Our body doesn't need that much junk. What are you feeling? What are you truly longing for?"

Feeling Self: "I feel bored and lonely. I want some excitement."

STEP 4: Reinforce the limit and reassure your *feeling self* that you are always there to take care of her and help meet her needs.

Inner Nurturer (as Inner Limit-Setter): "We do need to stop at one cookie and one scoop."

Inner Nurturer: "It's not food you're longing for, it's stimulation. I'm here, and I will help you find something exciting and stimulating. Let's go in the other room and do something engaging."

Feeling Self: "I feel lonely and would like to have more friends and a boyfriend. Weekends always feel lonely."

Inner Nurturer: "I know that we don't have either in our life right now. But you've got me for sure, and I can help.

Feeling Self: "I still want chocolate — can we get some just for tonight?"

Inner Nurturer (as Inner Limit-Setter): "No. We're not going to get any chocolate tonight."

Inner Nurturer: "Let's go home — we can have some fruit with peanut butter and sit on the couch and relax. Then together we can decide on some places we can go to try and meet new people."

Feeling Self: "Okay, but I'd rather have *chocolate* with peanut butter."

Feeling Self: "Wow, I love the way these shoes look. I want them."

Inner Nurturer (as Inner Limit-Setter): "They are way too expensive, and we need to stick to the budget and not spend any more money."

Feeling Self: "But it's hard to find shoes that fit, that I like, in this color. I want them! I need them!"

Inner Nurturer: "That may be true, but we really do have enough shoes. I'm sure we will find something similar when we can afford it. What does it feel like there isn't enough of?"

Feeling Self: "Feeling good about myself. I feel attractive in these shoes, and I don't feel very attractive lately."

Inner Nurturer: "You don't need new shoes to feel attractive. You are always beautiful and attractive. I love you just the way you are."

Inner Nurturer (as Inner Limit-Setter): "We're going to stick to our budget and not buy the shoes."

Inner Nurturer: "Let's go do something nurturing that doesn't involve spending money or eating.

Feeling Self: "All right, but I'd still like to have the shoes."

Setting Limits Means Delaying Gratification

M. Scott Peck, MD, author of *The Road Less Traveled*, defines delaying gratification as "a process of scheduling the pain and pleasure of life in such a way as to enhance the pleasure by meeting and experiencing the pain first and getting it over with."

Most children learn the skill of delaying gratification early in life, often by the time they begin school, at age five. Throughout childhood we have many opportunities to learn and practice this skill. We are told to eat our vegetables before we can have dessert. We'll have to finish our homework and chores before we can watch television. And we have to complete the school term before we can enjoy the carefree days of summer.

If our caregivers have mastered this skill, they reinforce our learning by leading disciplined lives and modeling restraint. They demonstrate patience and the willingness to persevere through the sacrifice and suffering inherent in child rearing. They delay buying things for themselves so we can get braces on our teeth and go to college. Perhaps they turn down career paths and promotions for the sake of the family.

By the time we reach adulthood, most of us have learned to consistently delay gratification to some extent. We study for and pass exams, go on to college, hold down jobs, manage our finances, pay our bills on time, and even raise children. So how is it that we can be disciplined in many areas of our lives and so undisciplined with respect to self-care, primarily eating and exercise? I have seen some of the most successful, disciplined individuals despair over their inability to stop overeating.

To the emotional eater, delaying gratification means enduring deprivation and tolerating uncomfortable cravings and impulses. It reminds us of a chronic experience of lack and limitation we seem to know well. We know the past, and there was *not enough* of a lot of things. We are not about to give up gratification in the present moment for some possible gratification or goal in the future. The future is sketchy, unknown, and unpredictable. What guarantee is there that delaying our gratification now will lead to fulfillment in the future? Sure, we may lose some weight, but at what price?

Your inability to apply the skill of delaying gratification to all areas of your life is a sign of imbalance. The root of this imbalance appears to be the quality of the nurturance you received as a child.

Peck suggests that the love our caregivers provide is even more important than their role-modeling behavior in our development of the skill of delaying gratification. "When we love something," he says, "it is of value to us, and when something is of value to us we spend time with it, time enjoying it and time taking care of it." Caregivers who devote time to the children they care for will take note of a child's need for discipline by observing the child's behaviors. They will observe the child's study, eating, play, problem solving, and even storytelling habits. They will gently assist their children in making the appropriate adjustments toward self-discipline.

The majority of emotional eaters have one thing in common: their childhoods did not feel predominantly nourishing. Even if their caregivers were kind and well intentioned, most emotional eaters did not receive the kind of dedicated, loving attention required to fully develop the self-care skill of delaying gratification.

The Ten-Minute Pause

You can learn to delay gratification even if you were not lucky enough to have been raised by loving, patient, self-disciplined caregivers or to have been born with a high tolerance for frustration. And you can do this with a timely pause.

When to pause: when you want to eat and you're not hungry; want to eat and you're already full; are hungry and want to indulge in unhealthy comfort food rather than making a healthy choice; want to impulsively spend money, use drugs or alcohol, sex, drama, and so on; or want to procrastinate.

What to do: STOP, slow down, and make the conscious choice to delay gratification for ten minutes and begin a Limit-Setting Inner Conversation.

Say to yourself: "I am willing to be uncomfortable for ten minutes so that I can reach my goals."

Remind yourself: I *can* endure discomfort for a short while. It's not root canal or childbirth!

Learning to delay gratification is a process that requires patience and practice. Your impulsive *feeling self* wears you down and gets you into trouble. Guiding her toward a more disciplined life has immense rewards. Each meal, purchase, or urge to procrastinate is a new opportunity to practice self-discipline.

Acknowledge and praise yourself for any success you have in delaying gratification. Remember to be proud of even the smallest step. The road to recovery is built on many of these tiny steps — many, many, many Limit-Setting Inner Conversations.

By regularly taking the time to connect with yourself in this way, you are creating a very nurturing inner world. And when your inner world feels consistently loving, safe, and secure, you can delay gratification when you need to, confident that whatever you're desiring will still be available later.

Setting Realistic Limits

Do you have a tendency to apply black-and-white thinking in your approach to limit setting? Starting tomorrow, you're going to *totally* stop eating sugary desserts, drinking diet sodas, and watching too much television? This is a surefire way to set up a *feeling-self* rebellion.

See if you can set a limit in the gray area. Try sugar-free desserts a few times per week. Or gradually taper off sugary desserts, diet sodas, or excessive television watching. There is no rush in setting limits, and the gradual approach helps to break the all-or-nothing mentality and ensure follow-through.

As a general rule, if you feel anxiety about a limit you're setting, or if the new limit is an extreme change from what you're already doing, it's probably not realistic. Most likely, you're trying to set an unrealistic limit because you want change *immediately*. You want to end the pain you are in *now*. You don't like slow progress, the kind that hardly makes a dent. But keep in mind that the process of changing long-term habits is a gradual one. It's all about progress, not perfection. And going slow allows you to practice delaying gratification over and over again.

"My Efforts Are Finally Paying Off"

A few months after making her list, Barbara made an important discovery.

I've been practicing my Inner Conversations regularly and journaling a couple of times a week. I've also been diligently working on reframing my negative self-talk. I'm really excited — it's all paying off, and I'm beginning to experience within myself a more loving, kind voice. And I feel more soothed by this voice.

I'm also feeling a lot more hopeful about my life. I feel better connected to the friends I have, and I've started dating again. I'm volunteering two times a month with a cat-rescue organization, and I'm happy to report that I'm getting lots of affection from a sweet little kitty I've named Hope.

And I've come to realize that my Inner Limit-Setter is truly an Inner Nurturer. I can trust her, because she's not the same as my harsh Inner Critic. Setting limits with myself is becoming easier, at times even effortless. I'm realizing that limits are actually nurturing and a form of self-care. They help me meet my goals. I'm noticing more willingness in myself and less resistance. This feels miraculous. Prior to this, I didn't believe I would ever stop overeating.

Setting Limits on Others

Just as we must learn to set limits for ourselves, we need to learn how to set limits, or boundaries, between ourselves and others. Personal boundaries are protective. They are psychological edges or limits that define where we end and the world or another begins. If they're effective, they keep us safe from harm while allowing us to take in what we need. If they are firm yet flexible, and not too loose or too rigid, they will allow in the warmth, connection, closeness, safety, and intimacy we need and desire.

We begin life within the body of another. Our earliest experiences with boundaries include a feeling of "boundary-less-ness." Mommy and I are one. Oneness is heavenly, blissful. Separation is terrifying. And yet the urge to separate and carve out a unique self appears to be programmed into our biology. As soon as we can crawl, we begin the journey. During the first three years of life, we slowly transition from oneness to separateness, from life without boundaries to a life full of boundaries. *This is mine. That's yours. It's okay to touch this. Don't touch that!* Throughout our childhood we test, define, retest, and redefine our boundaries.

If our caregivers model healthy, appropriate boundaries and encourage our growing autonomy, we feel entitled to have boundaries and comfortable asserting them. Caregivers with poor boundaries raise children with poor boundaries.

Loose Boundaries Lead to Merging

When our boundaries are too loose, we merge easily with the emotions and needs of others. We have little sense of our own separate self and difficulty identifying our emotions and needs. We feel confusion about who we are and what we want — often we present ourselves differently with different people. We may be hypersensitive to others' comments and criticisms and may personalize these to excess.

We tend to get overinvolved in other people's lives — we give too much and try too hard. We may try to fix or control others with our opinions, judgments, demands, and advice. While this may look and feel like care, it often unconsciously represents our own need for caretaking. We try to fix the people we are closest to so that we can then have *our own* needs met.

We may take on more work and outside commitment than is healthy for us. We may feel the need for constant connection with others and try to avoid being alone too much. When we are alone, we may feel lost, without direction, unmotivated, apathetic, empty, overwhelmed, and anxious or depressed.

Our loose boundaries represent an attempt to avoid the uncomfortable and terrifying feelings we associate with separateness and aloneness. While merging with others provides us with a sense of connection, purpose, and perhaps safety, it tends to disconnect us from ourselves. This disconnection leads us right back to eating for comfort and soothing.

"All I Want to Do Is Watch Television and Eat"

Sandra, a single, forty-eight-year-old, well-liked, and hardworking human resource manager, expressed this to me:

> I know my boundaries are way too loose. I get overinvolved in everyone else's life and need to focus more on what I want and need. But I find that when I'm alone, I can't motivate myself to work on personal goals. I feel kind of lost, unfocused, and overwhelmed. All I want to do is watch my favorite programs and eat. I'm there for my aging parents, and I worry constantly about my two older brothers and my best friend, who's surviving breast cancer. I'd like to have a boyfriend, but I'm afraid that having a man in my life will mean one more person to take care of.

Sandra has become disconnected from her own emotions and needs. Saying no to the constant requests of others makes her feel guilty, and she fears rejection. Taking care of the needs of others allows her to avoid these unpleasant emotions, but there's a price — she constantly feels drained. Too much aloneness evokes anxiety and overwhelms her. Eating, which is soothing and nurturing, brings about a heavenly, albeit temporary, *nondemanding* blissful experience of merging or oneness.

Rigid Boundaries Lead to Isolation

Our rigid boundaries represent an attempt to avoid the uncomfortable and often terrifying feeling of anxiety we associate with closeness. We don't let others get too close because intimacy is frightening. Too much closeness brings on a feeling of being suffocated or engulfed. We fear the loss of our separateness and independence. We may also avoid intimacy with ourselves and feel afraid of connecting to our inner world, where our harsh Inner Critic resides.

We may have a pattern of underinvolvement in work, community, and relationships, which can lead to emptiness and depression. Perhaps we don't know how to handle the constant intrusions others make into our lives. We may find it challenging to relate to the emotions and needs of others and may have difficulty giving and receiving care and concern. The downside is that others do not get to see who we truly are and all we have to offer.

While our rigid boundaries protect us, they can also leave us feeling chronically isolated and frustrated with the lack of nourishing relationships in our lives.

"I Feel So All Alone"

Jean, a top-notch insurance agent, was well aware that her boundaries were rigid. Divorced and living alone, she preferred it that way. Early on, Jean's parents had rejected their daughter's desire for closeness. Her parents were cold and aloof, and Jean, an only child, rarely experienced warmth, empathy, or compassion from them. She had consciously stopped wanting anything from them long ago. While this type of disconnection helped her survive a childhood full of neglect, she had trouble bonding with others, since she often couldn't relate to their emotions.

Jean had married a man like her father, who, she said, was "emotionally distant and cold." She tended to be attracted to men and women who were arrogant and aloof. Since her divorce, she had gained a large amount of weight and was concerned about her habit of consuming rich, fatty foods every night. "I'm sure my eating has something to do with the lack of intimacy and close friends in my life," she told me. "I know I need to allow others to get closer to me. But it seems that every time I do, it only results in misery. I guess I crave the closeness but also feel ambivalent about it."

Intimacy and connection require vulnerability, and vulnerability makes Jean feel unsafe and anxious. Eating, which is soothing and nurturing, brings about the nourishment and deliciousness of intimacy without the risk of hurt or loss.

Boundary Checklist: Evaluating Your Boundaries

This checklist will help you determine whether your boundaries are too loose, too rigid, or a combination of both. Try not to judge where you are at today. This is only a snapshot in time, and you can begin today to tighten or loosen your boundaries where appropriate.

The Boundary Checklist

Please check the statements that apply to you:

Loose Boundaries

❑ I often have difficulty identifying and expressing my own emotions and needs.

❑ I am often swayed by, or I accommodate, those more assertive than myself.

❑ Even though I often feel sensitive to or hurt by the comments of others, I can share my emotions easily.

❑ I sometimes feel compelled to share too much about myself or others and then I later feel vulnerable, ashamed, or guilty.

❑ I can easily get overinvolved in other people's emotions, needs, and problems.

❑ I have difficulty allowing others to see who I truly am; often I'm not clear about who I am and I present myself as the person I think others want me to be.

❑ I sometimes feel like a different person with different people.

❑ I feel the need to be in constant contact with others; I don't like to be alone.

❑ If a relationship ends, I often feel responsible for it ending and feel anxious or depressed for a long while.

❑ If people don't like me, I often feel I must have done something to cause their dislike.

❑ I feel compelled to check telephone and email messages regularly.

Rigid Boundaries

❑ I often have difficulty identifying my own emotions and needs, although I tend to be more aware of anger, irritation, and frustration than other emotions.

❑ I can sometimes be aggressive rather than assertive and have difficulty accommodating the needs of others.

❑ I often feel sensitive to or hurt by the comments of others and so do not share my true emotions much.

❑ I think sometimes I deny having any emotions or needs.

❑ I tend to keep my emotions and thoughts to myself. When I do express them, they sometimes come out harsh or overly critical.

❑ I do not really enjoy hearing about other people's problems in depth, other than out of curiosity or comparison to myself.

❑ I prefer to put some distance between myself and the emotions and needs of others.

❑ I am the same person no matter who I am around.

❑ I think I fear exposure, rejection, shame, and being controlled.

❑ I tend to isolate myself and am often disappointed in others.

❑ If a relationship ends, I tend to blame the other person and then move on.

❑ I screen telephone calls and procrastinate about returning calls and emails. I don't like to talk or connect if I'm not in the mood.

Please circle the type of boundary that best fits you:

Overly loose   Both loose and rigid   Overly rigid

Adjusting Your Boundaries

Good news! You've already learned in the previous chapters all the skills you'll need in order to adjust your boundaries.

If your boundaries are too loose, the following steps will help you firm them up:

1. List all the areas where you have loose boundaries, and set a conscious intention to take action and firm up one area at a time. Remind yourself that setting boundaries is not *selfish* but an important form of self-care.

2. Practice identifying and expressing your emotions and needs (review self-care skill #1, in chapter 2), so that you can more clearly define a separate self. This way you can have the closeness you seek without the risk of losing your sense of self.

3. Practice identifying and replacing any negative, critical, judgmental, personalizing, and catastrophizing thoughts with positive, energizing reframes (review self-care skill #2, in chapter 3). A more positive inner world fosters intimacy without the hypersensitivity you've lived with for so long.

4. Access your Inner Nurturer and soothe and comfort yourself with loving, supportive phrases as you make boundary adjustments. This will help you tolerate any new unpleasant emotions and thoughts that surface when you tighten your boundaries and others react to your newly defined self.

Often when we adjust our boundaries, we transition from one set of unpleasant emotions to another. In the beginning, these new emotions don't feel as if they reinforce our new boundary-setting effort. For example, let's say you decide to set a boundary between yourself and your younger sister who calls you multiple times per day to share her problems. You're currently feeling both annoyed and drained by all the calls. You make a kind and loving request that she try to care for herself a bit more and not call you multiple times per day. You reassure her that you love and care for her and that you believe she can meet some of her needs on her own.

She reacts with anger, throws a tantrum, and hangs up on you. Now you feel guilt, hurt, and anger, and you fear there will be weeks of drama. A new set of unpleasant emotions to deal with! These were the emotions you were avoiding with your loose boundaries.

Do not capitulate and go back to excessive caretaking of your sister. Access your Inner Nurturer and use your wisdom to remind yourself that your sister is just overreacting. It may take a day, a week, or six months, but she will most likely come to her senses. You do not need to feel guilty, nor do you need to overcare for her. You are entitled to have personal boundaries, and she is not entitled to use you to avoid growing up. Remind yourself that you can tolerate these new, unpleasant emotions, *however long it takes*. This experience has offered you another opportunity to nurture yourself with nourishing boundaries *rather than food*.

If your boundaries are too rigid, the following steps will help you loosen them up:

1. Identify all the areas where you have rigid boundaries, and set a conscious intention to take action and loosen up one area at a time. Remind yourself that you can redefine your boundary and express yourself if others get too close or intrusive.

2. Practice identifying and expressing your emotions and needs (review self-care skill #1, in chapter 2) so that you can better connect to yourself and others. Your emotions are the signals that inform you whether an "other" feels safe and warm or unsafe.

3. Practice identifying and replacing any negative, critical, judgmental, personalizing, and catastrophizing thoughts with positive, energizing reframes (review self-care skill #2, in chapter 3). A more positive inner world makes it safe for us to invite closeness without the fear of exposure and risk of rejection. Holding positive thoughts about others and our ability to tolerate closeness makes us want to get closer.

4. Access your Inner Nurturer and nourish yourself with loving supportive phrases as you make boundary adjustments. This will help you tolerate the unpleasant emotions and thoughts that surface when you loosen your boundaries and others begin to come closer.

"Let Me Think about It and Get Back to You"

As Sandra began to take a closer look at her boundaries, she could see that she rarely said no to anyone. Because of her need for approval and acceptance, she tried hard to please *everyone*. In order to stop overeating and lose weight, she would have to please herself as well.

Sandra set the intention to take the time she needed to check in with herself and have an Inner Conversation *before* saying yes to others' requests. She realized that she needed to assert herself and state that she would get back to them with her decision. At first she found this to be very uncomfortable, and she worried how others would react. Her Inner Nurturer had to work overtime to reassure her that it was okay to have boundaries and to say no or, "Let me think about that and get back to you."

What surprised Sandra was that most people accepted her boundaries easily, without any fuss. Friends and family members encouraged her to take more time for herself. She realized that she had been overgiving, unnecessarily. While her new sense of separateness led to feelings of aloneness and a sense of "not being needed," she was able to remind herself that her *feeling self*, whom she had neglected for a long time, needed her the most.

"I'm Getting Better at Reading My Emotional Signals"

Jean knew that she gravitated toward emotionally unavailable men, but until we worked together she was unaware of how she truly felt in their presence. She set the intention to check in with herself more often; and as she did check in, she noticed that she actually felt invisible and lonely around aloof men. She also noticed that she had a tendency to "perform" around this type of man. She would stimulate conversation and show a lot of interest in an attempt to get approval and attention. This energized her and kept the focus off of her. She had become somewhat addicted to this kind of stimulation and arousal. Men who were kind and available seemed boring in comparison.

Jean was committed to changing this pattern; she wanted to stop chasing men who ultimately rejected her. When she met a new man, she checked in with her *feeling self* for that feeling of being invisible, lonely, and energized. If it was present, she then accessed her Inner Nurturer for a reminder that she should consider her own needs and that this type of guy was not good for her.

Jean made a conscious decision to go out with "nice" men; and even though she didn't feel the familiar sense of excitement, she did notice that she felt visible and cared for. Although she felt more vulnerable, she was also feeling more nourished by the company of kind, caring men.

She decided to loosen her boundaries and allow new, supportive female friends into her life as well. As she began to allow the good to flow in, she noticed that her late-night binges were diminishing.

Are You Ready to Feast on Self-Love?

Self-connection provides the foundation you'll need in order to tolerate the emotions that surface when you set limits on yourself and others. Experiencing a state of enough-ness makes limit-setting more tolerable. As you become more comfortable with setting limits and boundaries, you'll notice how truly nurturing they are and how they enable you to meet your needs and goals.

Now it's time to supercharge your self-care skills and strengthen the foundation you've already built by developing the four habits that self-loving people naturally engage in.

CHAPTER SIX

Skill #5. Practice Accepting and Loving Yourself Unconditionally

I am saddened when I hear the stream of negative, critical, unloving comments that clients, seminar attendees, and participants in my twelve-week program often verbalize about their bodies and selves.

"I can't love and accept myself *as is* with these thunderous thighs."
"I won't go out in public in a sleeveless shirt; I hate my fat, flabby arms."
"My calves are unattractive and stubby; I rarely wear dresses."
"My skin is scarred from acne; I can't make peace with it."
"I have no real chin and my face is moon shaped; I hate it."
"I dislike my passive, introverted nature; I wish I were an extrovert."
"I'm not the kind of woman men go for. I'm not sexy enough."
"I'm old and unattractive now; it's hopeless."
"I procrastinate on everything and am especially bad at managing my finances. What's to love about that?"

Your relationship with food will remain imbalanced as long as you continue to shame and reject yourself and your body. You will use food to soothe, nurture, distract, pleasure, and even punish yourself. My goal in this chapter is to help you reclaim and honor the parts of yourself that you have neglected, disowned, or even discarded.

Self-Love Begins with Self-Acceptance

It's easy for us to accept the traits we possess that we like or that others deem positive. We feel good about our witty sense of humor, our musical ability, our sharp intellect, and our level of empathy and compassion for others. Most of us have some aspects of our body that we appreciate and view with positive regard. We love our thick head of hair. We like our smile and our straight teeth. We've been told we have a great derriere.

It's difficult, however, for most of us to accept our excess body fat, double chin, cellulite, acne, and body parts we believe to be too big, too small, or out of proportion. We may wish we were smarter, funnier, younger, more driven, entrepreneurial, or athletic and find it hard to accept the areas where we believe we fall short. We long to have been born with different genetics. We compare ourselves to and envy those who have the traits and bodies we would like to have. We find it challenging to accept and love ourselves unconditionally — flaws, bulges, inadequacies, scars, and all. It seems nearly impossible to stop regularly disparaging ourselves with critical comments and judgments.

When we receive consistent parental love and care, we enter adulthood with a solidly internalized sense of value and worth. Loving ourselves and others comes easy. We naturally gravitate toward people and situations that mirror our positive sense of self.

If our caregivers and family members devalue or negate themselves or us, we learn to do the same. When we observe and are raised with unreasonable expectations, unfair comparisons, excessive criticism, judgment, or humiliation, we experience and internalize a sense of shame and unworthiness. We learn to reject and diminish ourselves because we experienced rejection in place of loving-kindness, acceptance, and validation.

Unconditional self-acceptance is at the core of loving ourselves.

Albert Ellis, PhD, founder of Rational Emotive Behavior Therapy and coauthor of *The Secret of Overcoming Verbal Abuse*, suggests we adopt a philosophy of unconditional self-acceptance, one that, I believe, gets to the heart of the matter: "I will always define myself as a good or worthy individual — just because I exist, just because I am alive, just because I am human. I will not rate anything."

This means that you are *always* worthy and acceptable even though your body isn't perfect and you've made mistakes, achieved less than you'd hoped to, performed poorly, acted badly, and so on. You don't think less of yourself as a person because of what you look like, do, have, or have done. You don't rate yourself as unworthy because you have body parts that don't measure up to the culturally defined notions of beauty. You don't rate yourself as unacceptable because you have a passive personality or are an introvert or because your IQ is not above 140.

You may experience remorse, regret, or even sadness for yourself or your behavior, but this doesn't diminish your worth. You accept the responsibility for and consequences of your actions and make apologies when appropriate, but you do not rate your entire being as bad because something you did was not right.

You unconditionally accept your body size, body parts, personality traits, and perceived flaws today, as they are. This doesn't mean you wouldn't prefer to have been born with a different body or attributes. Nor does it mean you can't seek to improve yourself.

Loving yourself unconditionally means *accepting yourself without conditions*. You acknowledge and embrace who you are, what you look like, where you are in your life, and where you have been. Why is it so important to accept yourself unconditionally? After all, wouldn't self-acceptance give you license to keep overeating and to stay on the couch watching television all day? Doesn't self-acceptance represent resignation, a sort of giving up and giving in to your own mediocrity?

Actually, the opposite is true. Self-acceptance does not represent resignation because it is not a matter of *giving up*. Rather, it is an act of *giving to*. You give to yourself the gift of compassion, which is at the core of any loving relationship. You *give* to yourself the developmentally significant acceptance and validation that you did not receive enough of as a child.

Self-Rejection Leads to Overeating

Self-rejection and -condemnation trigger both hopelessness and power-lessness. These states are not motivating, and they lead to depression, loneliness, apathy, resignation, isolation, and emotional eating. When we lack self-love, we keep ourselves imprisoned by the images and senses we have of ourselves and our bodies. We regularly compare ourselves to others and unreasonable societal standards. By constantly recycling any negative self-commentary and focusing on critical comments made by others, we deny ourselves the love and kindness that is our birthright.

When we have not learned to love ourselves, we regularly look out-side for validation and approval. Just as water seeks its own level, we gravitate toward others who mirror back to us their own low self-esteem and poor self-acceptance, even though they may appear confident. Their energy feels familiar to us; it resonates with what we have come to believe about ourselves.

Someone told you long ago that you were unworthy of love; you were not acceptable because you were too much of this or too little of that. You were told you were "too sensitive," "too serious," "too fat," "too short," "too tall," or "too smart." You were told you were "not pretty enough," "not outgoing enough," or "not athletic enough." I remember my mother telling me over and over in my late teens and early twenties that I was "too smart" and that I shouldn't be so smart because "men don't like smart women." I wanted to strangle her every time she said it.

Your self-rejection stems from the discrepancy between who you would like to be and who you are. You have waged a cruel and destructive war within, splitting yourself into good and bad parts.

Unrealistic societal standards have objectified you and minimized your sense of your innate worth. Constant rejection and shame have led you to believe that you are inadequate as you are; that you are defec-tive, flawed, and not lovable, perhaps beyond repair. You've been led to believe that it is best to hide or cover up certain body parts and personal-ity traits.

Loving yourself in a culture filled with unrealistic standards of beauty, personality, and success requires courage. It is ultimately an act of separation and individuation, demanding boldness and even rebellion. You must refuse to collude with narrowly defined cultural notions of attractiveness, accomplishment, and worthiness. You'll need to expand your definition of beauty to include all shapes, colors, sizes, and ages. And you'll need to broaden your definition of success to encompass many paths and accomplishments, big and small.

When we can acknowledge and enjoy our strengths and compassionately honor and embrace our weaknesses, we begin to see ourselves as the sum of our parts, a unique and worthwhile whole. This loving inner environment, free of contempt and self-rejection, sets the stage for further personal growth and transformation. Our willingness to shift and change emerges, and our long-held resistance begins to recede. We stop wasting precious time and energy hating ourselves and our bodies. We stop resisting and start accepting what is. We set ourselves free to pursue self-improvement, productivity, or creative projects. And we form more loving alliances with those around us as our self-acceptance and self-love translate into greater acceptance of others.

How Accepting Are You of Yourself?

Complete the Self-Acceptance Questionnaire on pages 122–23 to get an idea of your level of self-acceptance today. This will help you identify which habits you already have in place and which ones you'll need to develop.

The Four Habits You Must Develop

Learning to love and accept yourself is a process; all that is required is the willingness to practice. You can unlearn self-rejection and gently move toward self-love and acceptance by developing the habits that people with a healthy level of self-acceptance naturally engage in. These four habits are as follows:

Self-Acceptance Questionnaire

For each trio of statements, choose the letter (*a*, *b*, or *c*) that is most true for you, and circle the corresponding *X*.	HIGH	MODERATE	LOW
1a. I regularly appreciate and acknowledge my strengths and accomplishments, big and small.	X		
1b. I sometimes appreciate and acknowledge my strengths and accomplishments, big and small.		X	
1c. I tend to minimize or ignore my strengths and accomplishments.			X
2a. I honor and embrace my weaknesses, imperfections, and inadequacies.	X		
2b. I can embrace some aspects and I struggle with embracing others.		X	
2c. I tend to split myself into good and bad parts and focus mainly on the bad.			X
3a. I practice compassion with myself and speak lovingly to myself most of the time.	X		
3b. I can be kind to myself at times, but I can also be harsh with myself.		X	
3c. I regularly criticize and judge myself. Self-compassion feels awkward and unnatural.			X
4a. I believe I am worthy of love, and I love myself unconditionally.	X		
4b. I sometimes feel worthy, but at other times I feel very unworthy. I have difficulty with unconditional self-love.		X	
4c. Intellectually, I know I'm worthy of love. But emotionally, I just don't feel it.			X
5a. In general, my expectations of myself and my body are reasonable.	X		
5b. Some of my expectations are reasonable, some are too high, and some are too low.		X	
5c. My expectations tend to be either too high or too low.			X
6a. I make a point *not* to use *should*s with myself or others.	X		
6b. I sometimes fall prey to the "tyranny of the *should*s."		X	
6c. I use the *should* word often.			X

Self-Acceptance Questionnaire

	HIGH	MODERATE	LOW
7a. I focus my attention on aspects of my life I *can* change. I don't waste time focusing on things I can't change.	X		
7b. I focus somewhat on aspects I'd like to change, but I must admit I spend too much time lamenting things I can't change.		X	
7c. I don't think about change much — I don't like change. I dislike so much about myself and my life that I often feel hopeless. I often wish I were someone else or that I didn't exist.			X
8a. When I compare myself to others, I use the comparison for inspiration and motivation.	X		
8b. I try not to compare myself, but I do get caught up in envying what others have and feeling bad about myself.		X	
8c. I compare myself to others often. Sometimes I win the comparison; other times I lose. I struggle with jealousy.			X
9a. I consciously practice forgiving myself for perceived mistakes and failures.	X		
9b. I can forgive myself for some things but definitely have things I just can't seem to forgive myself for.		X	
9c. I don't forgive myself for many things. I'm not sure I believe in forgiveness or am capable of it.			X
10a. I consciously set aside time to grieve losses and disappointments. I know how valuable grieving is.	X		
10b. I do some grieving when I feel sad, but I don't make a point to set aside time to grieve. It's unpleasant.		X	
10c. I rarely grieve anything.			X
My overall level of self-acceptance is: Circle the level that represents the greatest number of circled Xs.	HIGH	MODERATE	LOW

Habit 1. Practice self-affirming commentary and dialogues.

Habit 2. Adjust your expectations. Be realistic about what you can change or achieve.

Habit 3. Use comparisons for inspiration and motivation only.

Habit 4. Forgive yourself for perceived mistakes and failures.

Habit 1. Practice Self-Affirming Commentary and Dialogues

Unconditional self-acceptance translates into daily self-talk that is positive and affirmative. We accentuate our strengths and accomplishments, large and small, and compassionately embrace our weaknesses, shortcomings, and mistakes. When we have self-denigrating thoughts, we catch them quickly and replace them with energizing reframes.

Self-affirming commentary consists of statements you make to yourself that are unconditionally supportive and positive. No matter what a situation entails, you *always* support and encourage yourself. You can practice this by praising yourself every day for small accomplishments and speaking to yourself with kindness when you are disappointed in yourself.

Examples of self-affirming commentary:

"I'm proud of myself for clearing out the garage today."

"I like the way I handled that phone call."

"Although I didn't score well on the exam, I give myself A for effort. I'll do better next time."

"I exercised once this week; that's great, it's more than zero."

"It's all right that my skin looks blotchy tonight. I'm so much more than my skin, and people relate to me as a whole package."

"These clothes are tight — I must have gained some weight. I'll put on looser clothes because I deserve to be comfortable. Tonight when I get home I'll figure out a few small dietary changes I can make — I'll get the weight back off!"

Handling the "Yes, Buts"

Your *feeling self* may not feel that she is worthy of love and acceptance the way she is, and she may retort with a "yes, but..." when you say loving phrases to her. At these times, you'll need your Inner Nurturer to step in, reaffirm that you *are* worthy of kindness and compassion, and offer some wisdom regarding the situation.

It can be helpful when you're learning self-love and acceptance to hear the words and phrases of compassionate loving beings. The more exposure you have to others who are unconditionally loving, the easier it will be for you to learn and practice self-love. In individual or group psychotherapy, I often play the role of the Inner Nurturer so that clients can hear the language of love. For some, it's the first time they have experienced unconditional acceptance, and it feels nourishing *and* foreign.

"I Dislike My Shy Personality"

This is a self-affirming dialogue I role-played with Jan, a sweet, quiet, and lovely nurse-practitioner:

Jan: "I dislike my shy, introverted personality. It makes socializing excruciatingly painful."

Julie (as Jan's Inner Nurturer): "I love you, Jan, just the way you are. You are very sensitive, intuitive, and perceptive, and these are wonderful qualities."

Jan: "Yes, but I don't do well in large parties or crowds. I'm very uncomfortable."

Julie: "We are all born with personality types best suited to certain social settings. Your quiet, reflective personality is a gift, and it's best suited to intimate gatherings."

Jan: "I guess it's okay for me to stick with gatherings that suit my personality and stop trying to be something I'm not."

Julie: "Absolutely."

"It's *Not* Okay to Make a Mistake"

I role-played this self-affirming dialogue with Tess, a conscientious web designer in a large advertising firm:

Tess: "I can't believe I made such a big, stupid mistake. It could cost me my job."

Julie (as Tess's Inner Nurturer): "It's okay to make a mistake. You're human. I love and value you even when you make mistakes."

Tess: "Yes, but it's *not* okay to make a careless, ridiculous, stupid mistake like I made."

Julie: "Even caring, wonderful, hardworking, dedicated people make careless mistakes. It is not possible to be perfect. Constantly beating yourself up will be mistake number two. Let's take a lesson from this and get clear on what we can do to be more careful in the future."

Tess: "Okay. You're right. I am hardworking and dedicated and will never be perfect. I'm being too hard on myself. And I know what I can do differently next time."

"I HATE MY BIG FAT LEGS"

Here's a self-affirming dialogue I role-played with Theresa, a tireless mother of three children under the age of five:

Theresa: "I hate my big fat legs. I wish I had long, thin legs like my sister. There is just no way that I'm ever going to love these legs."

Julie (as Theresa's Inner Nurturer): "To me, you are always beautiful, whole, and complete. I love and accept you just as you are."

Theresa: "Yes, but I don't believe that. My legs are big and fat and ugly, and people judge me for them. They are unsightly and full of cellulite. They are not beautiful. I hate them and always will."

Julie: "You don't have to have perfect body parts to be beautiful or lovable. Beauty emanates from the inside. You must expand your definition of beauty. Beauty comes in many sizes, shapes, and colors. You have given birth to three incredible children. Your legs are perfectly suited to do what they are meant to do: carry you through life and help you take care of these precious little ones. Anyone who judges you so harshly is not worth knowing. The fact that other people are incapable of loving behavior has nothing to do with you. I know that the judgment you've experienced regarding the size of your legs has been painful. Let's set aside some time to grieve this."

Theresa: "It's true, I'm sad that I've been made to feel that my legs don't measure up. And I can see that I'm my own harshest critic. I need to start practicing loving and accepting myself as I am. I am a woman and a mother, and the truth is, my body has served me well."

You may need to set aside time to grieve any disappointments or losses highlighted during your self-affirming dialogues. This will allow you to release any pent-up emotions, integrate the loss, and move toward greater self-acceptance. You may need to grieve a particular issue many times before you come to some level of acceptance.

It takes time to shift deeply held beliefs about yourself and your body. You may not feel better immediately after a self-affirming dialogue. It's the consistent practice of self-affirming commentary and dialogues, plus exposure to loving others, that will transform your perception of yourself, your body, and your life and reduce your emotional eating.

Habit 2. Adjust Your Expectations; Be Realistic about What You Can Change or Achieve

For most of us, there is a perceived gap between who we are and who we would like to be. Often our expectations of what we can and cannot achieve are unrealistic. Unrealistic expectations lead to what psychiatrist Karen Horney called "the tyranny of the *should*s." Your expectations are too high, too rigid, and too difficult to achieve, yet you believe you can and *should* achieve this vision of your idealized self. Often the *should*s are accompanied by a tendency to minimize what you *have* accomplished. "I *only* lost five pounds; I *should* have lost more."

Dr. Horney suggested there is a "disregard for feasibility": even when you see you cannot achieve these goals and meet your expectations, you still believe you *should* be able to, and that nothing *should* be impossible. Similarly, when we have low expectations, we believe we *should* be capable of more. This constant gap between what we expect of ourselves and what we are capable of doing highlights our lack of self-acceptance. It leads to self-rejection, disappointment, frustration, and emotional eating.

Can you relate to any of the following *should*s?

"I *should* be able to lose two pounds per week until summer."

"I *should* be able to stick to a restrictive eating plan — other people do."

"I *should* try to get down to a size six even though I don't think I have the genetics for it."

"I *should* be able to do the same amount of exercise I did years ago."

"I *should* have thinner thighs; I must not be working out enough."

"I *should* be able to control my food intake at all times."

"I *should* never show anger or frustration."

"I *should* not let anyone see me cry; it's a sign of weakness."

"I *should* always be kind, understanding, and polite."

ADJUSTING YOUR EXPECTATIONS

Our expectations of ourselves, situations, or other people can be too high, too low, or "just right" and reasonable. Of course, there are times when even low or high expectations can be reasonable. It would be reasonable for us to set our expectations low with respect to winning the lottery. On the other hand, high expectations may be very motivating for an athletic competition.

Most of us rarely check in with ourselves and explore what we expect from either ourselves or a given situation. If our life feels in balance, our expectations are most likely reasonable. It is generally when we feel a sense of disappointment, anger, frustration, or sadness that our unstated or unconscious expectations come to the foreground. This is the time to get clear on your expectations and adjust them if necessary. Just as you have learned to tune in and identify your self-defeating thoughts and core beliefs, you'll need to do the same with your expectations. You'll need to make them conscious and ask yourself if they are reasonable.

When our expectations are too low, we may feel disappointed in ourselves and our lives. Adjusting our expectations by setting them higher may leave us feeling anxious, overwhelmed, or pressured. We will have to tolerate these new unfamiliar emotions in order to accomplish more and actualize our potential.

Conversely, when our expectations are too high, we feel constant harsh pressure to do more or be more. We criticize and judge ourselves for not meeting our expectations. Perhaps we expect too much of others as well and are often disappointed in their behavior. Adjusting our expectations by lowering them a bit may leave us feeling inadequate, unexceptional, ordinary, disappointed, and less motivated. Tolerating these uncomfortable emotional states will help us find balance.

Is It Possible to Have Both High and Low Expectations?

Yes. My client Sherry, a psychologist for a large mental health agency, found that as a child, she could satisfy her parents' high expectations by getting good grades and honors and having a very active social life. But she was never able to meet their expectations about her body size. Today her expectations of herself regarding work and social obligations are very high, but her expectations about her self-care are very low. Sherry shared this with me:

> I expect to excel at work most of the time, and I do. I also have a busy social life, and I stay well connected with friends and family. It's also important to me to be a good daughter, wife, and friend. But when I drive myself that hard, I then feel it's okay to play hard; and that means eat and drink anything I want. I guess what I'm realizing is that my expectations may be too high when it comes to work, social, and familial obligations. I can't drive myself that hard to be perfect

without repercussions. I think I expect that I can handle it all, but the truth is I rebel with food.

"I'm Not Sure I Know What a Reasonable Expectation Is"

When I first began to work with Karen, she shared two major complaints. She was dissatisfied with both her weight and the significant relationships in her life. Her husband drank too much, and her brother, who lived three thousand miles away, was "negative and depressing." She described her few girlfriends as "self-absorbed and needy," and she rarely felt nourished by their company. She spent much of her time alone, reading and overeating.

It was clear to Karen that what she needed was more emotional intimacy and the feeling that the people in her life wanted to take the time to care for and listen to her. She was chronically disappointed by her husband's alcoholism and expected that at some point he would seek recovery. She thought that if she "gave enough" to the people in her life, they would reciprocate with the love and nurturance she needed. But because Karen had never experienced nourishing love in her family of origin, she had attracted people into her life who were familiar, or family-like: distant, self-focused, and emotionally immature. She wasn't sure if any of her expectations were reasonable.

I assured Karen that it was normal, healthy, and reasonable to need and desire emotional intimacy and care but that it might not be reasonable to expect it from people who are not capable of it. With a little support, Karen gathered the courage to find out whether her expectations were reasonable. She decided to ask her husband to attend couples counseling with her, because she felt he *was* capable of intimacy and that it was reasonable to expect him to try a little harder. She hoped that in couples counseling they could explore his drinking problem.

We examined her expectation that giving *more* to her friends or her brother would get her what she needed. She could see that this expectation was unreasonable and had left her feeling depleted and empty. She realized that she would have to attract new friends, because it was not reasonable to expect that her closest friends would change.

When we adjust our expectations to a reasonable level, we create emotional balance. We accept ourselves and others *as is*. We accept what we are capable of as well as what those closest to us are capable of. We free up our energy, in this moment, to focus on aspects of our lives that we can and choose to change.

It may be helpful to share your expectations with a trusted friend, mentor, or therapist. This can be a good way to find out how reasonable they are. Your best guide over time, however, will be how emotionally balanced you feel. If you expect something and the expectation is generally met without much struggle or strain, consider it reasonable. If your expectations are rarely met, or met only with lots of effort or heartache, they're probably not reasonable.

Habit 3. Use Comparisons for Inspiration and Motivation Only

We all compare ourselves to others. We do it automatically. We compare ourselves on many fronts: our body size and shape, attractiveness, youthfulness, accomplishments, possessions, and even relationships. We learn at an early age to compare ourselves to others as we observe caregivers, extended family members, and mentors making comparisons.

"You are just as smart and pretty as your sister."
"I can see you are not as athletic as Tommy."
"Penny got an A in English. Why are you getting only a B?"

Comparisons don't present a problem if they are self- and other-affirming and used to inspire and motivate:

"Wow, what a great guitar player Josh is. I hope to play that well someday."
"Look at how fit she is. I'd like to be that fit, and she motivates me to work out harder."
"I love her style. She inspires me to take the time to put together outfits."

Comparisons work best when they are win-win. The problem arises when we make comparisons in such a way that someone wins and someone loses. When we experience jealousy or envy, we often feel hopeless about our prospects of looking or being like someone or acquiring or achieving what they have. We make ourselves miserable with a series of thoughts that goes something like this:

Comparison thought: "*Oh my God*, she has an incredible figure. I could never look like that."

Self-rejecting thought: "I'm just a fat, dumpy, ugly blob. Who would ever love me with my body?"

Discounting-other-person thought: "She doesn't deserve to get so much attention just because she was born beautiful. She's probably shallow and superficial. I hate women like her, and I hate this culture."

Resultant emotions: Discouraged, depressed, frustrated, agitated, helpless, hopeless, angry, sad, jealous, and vindictive.

Comparison thought: "Wow, she must be supersuccessful or married to a rich guy to have an incredible home like this. Or maybe she inherited a lot of money. John and I will never make that kind of money, inherit money, or have a beautiful home."

Self-rejecting thought: "I picked the wrong career and married the wrong guy. I've never been good at figuring out how to get ahead in life."

Discounting-other-person thought: "If she didn't inherit money, she's probably a corporate-ladder climber or married to one. You've got to be ruthless and cutthroat to make that kind of money."

Resultant emotions: Powerless, frustrated, invisible, angry, sad, and jealous.

Comparisons can also be problematic when we use them to boost our own flagging self-esteem at someone else's expense.

Comparison thought: "I look much better than she does."

Self-affirming thought: "I may be overweight, but at least I haven't lost all control like her."

Discounting-other-person thought: "Boy, she is really heavy. She must binge all the time. That's pathetic."

Resultant emotions: Empowered, uplifted, encouraged.

This is not an effective way to resolve low self-esteem and put an end to self-rejection. It creates a temporary feel-good sensation but does not heal the deeper wounds. Nor does it promote self-acceptance, compassion, and empathy for ourselves and others. We seek out people whom we deem *less than* us in order to feel good about ourselves. We have to avoid people who trigger our jealousy, because they fuel our self-rejection and low self-esteem.

Comparing yourself to others in a win-lose way is often nothing more than a deeply ingrained bad habit. You can begin to break the habit with the realization that you are on your own unique path. You are not in competition with anyone. Your goal is to be the best possible version of *you*. Despite any illusion of scarcity and lack, there is truly enough good to go around. Accepting and honoring yourself and others unconditionally increases the good all around you.

When you observe others with attributes, bodies, accomplishments, families, friends, or things you wish you had, make the choice to try any of the following:

- Drop the habit of making *any* comparison to yourself; just notice whatever it is you like or admire about the others.
- Be generous of spirit; it will come back to you tenfold.
- Be happy for them and, in your mind, wish them well, as difficult as this may be — "fake it until you make it."
- Make the phrase "You go, girl/guy" your motto.
- Be inspired and motivated by the others if possible.
- View their beauty as you would artwork that you admire.
- View their accomplishments with respect, as you would those of a Nobel Prize winner.

- Remind yourself that you are not in competition with anyone and that you are more than your perceived inadequacies or flaws — you are a whole package.
- Remind yourself of all that you already have.
- Catch any self-rejecting comparison thoughts and replace them with self-affirming, self-esteem-enhancing, energizing reframes.
- Use self-affirming commentary and dialogues to practice self-love and self-acceptance.

Habit 4. Forgive Yourself for Perceived Mistakes and Failures

Continuing to beat yourself up for your mistakes is just plain unproductive. Self-acceptance demands compassion, and that means forgiveness. Like everything else, forgiveness is a process. It begins with allowing yourself to experience and express the emotions regarding the perceived mistake or failure. There is no rush in this process. Perhaps you regret not giving your best in a relationship, and you can't get that relationship back. Or you didn't take the best care of yourself and have been diagnosed with a serious medical condition. In both cases, you feel sad and ashamed. Most likely you were doing the best you could at the time. Expecting that you *should* have done better, and then beating yourself up, keeps you stuck in purgatory and fuels your emotional appetite.

Self-forgiveness means you adjust your expectations of yourself and you compassionately make room for error. There are always reasons why we behave the way we do. Sometimes when we find we cannot yet forgive ourselves, it may be because we still need to grieve the losses or disappointments associated with the mistake or failure.

Many emotional eaters I work with find it hard to forgive themselves for gaining large amounts of weight, for distorting and creating disease in their bodies, and for losing precious years to depression and anxiety. When I remind them that they came from dysfunctional families and entered adulthood with few self-care skills, they begin to grieve for the neglected, abandoned child that they were. They find it easier to forgive themselves when they realize that they were doing the best they could.

Take some time to explore the reasons you have for not forgiving yourself. In your journal, make a list of the things you haven't forgiven yourself for. Next to each item, write "I forgive myself completely." What comes up when you write this? Can you forgive yourself and let it go? What do you fear would happen if you forgave yourself? How would your life be different? Forgiving yourself may not take away the sadness you feel about something, but it's an important part of healing.

As strange as it may sound, not forgiving yourself may be a way to stay childlike, a way of not having to grow up and get on with your life. It may be a way to stay attached to the past and avoid uncomfortable forward movement. Forgiving yourself and others is an adult, mature act; it involves letting go of the past and moving on.

Healing a Poor Body Image or Self-Image

Practicing the four habits that foster self-acceptance is a good starting point for healing a poor body image or self-image. As emotional eaters, many of us have never truly felt at home with ourselves or in our own bodies. We have spent most of our lives feeling self-conscious and focusing on what's wrong with us. We have, in many ways, been unable to actualize our potential because we have lived for so long in a foggy, disconnected state of self-rejection and disgust.

If you have spent a good portion of your life feeling ashamed and insecure about your body or self, you may need additional psychotherapeutic work to help you heal the wounds and shift the beliefs and attitudes that block you from accepting and loving yourself. In addition to traditional talk therapy, there are a number of therapeutic techniques and modalities that can be helpful for healing painfully negative or distorted body images and self-images. While it's beyond the scope of this book to cover these techniques in depth, I include here a brief description of a few I find particularly helpful. These are healing-parts dialogues, guided imagery, mirror work, and dance/movement therapy. In my clinical practice, I have found all of these techniques to be effective for different people.

Healing-Parts Dialogues

I use a process I call healing-parts dialogues to help clients gain perspective and even gratitude for certain aspects of themselves that they dislike. The dialogues lead to a deeper therapeutic exploration of the disconnection from self, and they help to heal shame and move a person toward greater self-acceptance. I ask clients to dialogue with the body part, trait, or perceived flaw they dislike. The goal is to go back and forth, talking to a body part until the client comes to some level of acceptance, even if temporary. You may need to have a healing dialogue many times before you are ready to more fully accept that aspect of yourself. Here's an example:

> Cheryl: "Hello, big belly. I hate you. You're huge and you make me feel super-self-conscious. You don't fit well in clothes, you stick out, and you're not attractive. No matter what I do, I can't shrink you."
>
> Cheryl's belly: "Hello Cheryl. I'm the soft, flexible, curvy part of you that shrinks or expands depending on how you care for me. I know you wish I were smaller. But lately, you've been filling me up with a lot of food and negativity. How about feeding me more love and kindness?"
>
> Cheryl: "Well, it's hard for me to say nice things to you when you're this size. But the truth is, hating you makes me want to binge. And that's just a vicious cycle."
>
> Cheryl's belly: "Big or small, I'm here to support you.
>
> Cheryl: "Yeah, you're here to support me, and I'm totally unsupportive of you. I think I need to start appreciating all you do for me."
>
> Cheryl's belly: "Amen."

Guided Imagery

Guided imagery is a gentle yet powerful mind-body process that has been used for decades for relaxation, stress reduction, and emotional healing. The therapist uses a series of verbal suggestions to guide you in imagining experiences and sensations. By engaging in this right-brained activity, you're better able to regulate your emotions and access your intuition, creativity, abstract thinking, and empathy.

Mirror Work

I first learned of mirror work by reading Susie Orbach's book *Fat Is a Feminist Issue*. She writes:

> Most compulsive eaters are very aware of how their faces look but not in relation to the rest of their bodies. What we try to do in this exercise is to observe our bodies. We are using the mirror to see ourselves without judging the image it holds. This is both a frightening and [a] difficult project for many women because one is so used to making a grimace and judgment on the few occasions we do see our whole bodies. We are so familiar with avoiding possibly unacceptable visions, keeping our heads down as we walk past shop windows lest we cast a glance at ourselves unaware and trigger negative feelings.

The goal of mirror work is to be able to observe yourself without judgment and move toward greater self-acceptance and self-respect. Utilizing a full-length, undistorted mirror, you set aside time to observe, imagine, and, over time, transform your body image.

Dance/Movement Therapy

This is a psychotherapeutic modality utilizing movement to access emotions, sensations, thoughts, and stored memories to facilitate healing. It can be an effective way of accessing preverbal (before you could speak) feelings and sensations. I am not a dance/movement therapist, but I have referred clients to such therapists with good results. The American Dance Therapy Association is a good resource for finding a practitioner in your area.

Loving Yourself Thin

You began using food long ago to compensate for the acceptance, love, and nurturance missing from your life. Now as an adult, you can and must choose to love and accept yourself unconditionally and nurture yourself in nonfood ways. You don't need to wait until tomorrow, when you will lose the weight, get your face lifted, find a boyfriend, or land a better job. Loving yourself means giving yourself the support, kindness, and compassion you need and deserve *today*.

PART TWO

Tuning Up Biochemistry

CHAPTER SEVEN

When Overeating Is Driven by Body Imbalance

Your body comes equipped with an incredibly sophisticated signaling system designed to guide you in obtaining proper nutrition. The system informs you, via hunger pangs, that it's time to eat and prods you with cravings to select the nutrients needed. It calculates the caloric density of what you eat to ensure you get enough calories and then signals you when you're full. Just like breathing, most of these complex processes occur without your awareness. If you don't mess with the machinery too much, it will work well for a lifetime.

When we are infants and small children, our eating is intuitive and our signals are usually loud and clear. We eat when we're hungry and stop before we're full. We gravitate toward certain foods and avoid those we dislike. Animals in the wild exhibit this natural way of eating as well. Their internal signals guide them, and they effortlessly maintain their weight within an optimum range. There are also many examples of lean, healthy, long-living cultures around the globe that still exhibit this intuitive eating style. They don't count calories or weigh and measure food; they rely on their bodies to do these behind-the-scenes calculations.

As an emotional eater, you're most likely somewhat disconnected from your body signals. You've lost touch with your innate signaling system and often ignore, medicate, or override your body's messages.

Perhaps you've spent years living in a poorly functioning body, coping with unpleasant symptoms like digestive problems, bloating, and fatigue and with chronic inflammation such as headaches and joint pain.

You may be experiencing significant health warnings such as high blood sugar and blood pressure or may already have degenerative conditions like diabetes and heart disease.

Losing Touch with Our Signals

In part 1, I explained how unmet emotional needs can lead to disconnection from ourselves and our most basic *mind* signals, resulting in an emotional appetite and an exaggerated craving for pleasure, comfort, and soothing. Similarly, unmet or ignored bodily needs for things like proper nutrition, exercise, rest, and sleep can throw off our signaling system and disconnect us from our basic *body* signals. The result can be dulled hunger cues; an appetite that, once triggered, doesn't seem to shut off; intense and unrelenting food cravings; overeating; weight gain; fatigue; and a multitude of health problems.

How did we get so disconnected from our body signals? We live in a land of plenty — how is it that we can have unmet bodily needs? In this part of the book, I discuss the six major factors that contribute to this disconnection:

1. Cultural and family messages have encouraged us to ignore body signals in an attempt to control our body size, leading to a destructive diet mentality.
2. Chronic low-calorie dieting imbalances our signals and leads to dietary deficiencies, a slower metabolism, out-of-control rebound eating, and weight gain.
3. Our calorie-counting machinery gets fooled and thrown off by a modern diet artificially concentrated in fat, sugar, fiber-deficient processed foods, and foods of animal origin, including meat, fowl, fish, eggs, and dairy products. Obesity is on the rise because our diet has become substantially different from that of our ancestors.

4. Modern drug-like foods activate pleasure centers in the brain, unbalance body and brain signals, and lead to addiction. Once we're addicted, it takes a disciplined effort to tolerate the unpleasant process of detoxification and the reintroduction of less stimulating whole foods.

5. Genetics and lifestyle can cause body and brain conditions including hormonal irregularities, low or high levels of brain chemicals, and food allergies or sensitivities that result in imbalanced signals.

6. High-stress, 24/7, overstimulating, sedentary urban lifestyles downplay the need for proper exercise, rest, and sleep.

The Diet Mentality Is Hard to Break

I don't need to tell you that we live in a diet-obsessed culture. Americans spend over $65 billion a year on weight loss products and services. More that 100 million Americans are regular dieters, in spite of the fact that research demonstrates that 98 percent of all dieters regain their weight within five years, and 95 percent within two years.

When I use the term *diet mentality*, I am referring to deeply entrenched thoughts and habits related to controlling food intake and body size. See if any of these examples of the diet mentality apply to you:

- You constantly think about what you've eaten, what you'll eat, and what diet you're going to follow to lose weight.
- You regularly count and restrict calories, carbohydrates, and/or fat grams.
- You eat according to rules rather than body hunger — for example, you don't eat past a certain time of night and you fast, undereat, or skip meals when you feel fat or after you've overeaten.
- You avoid activities that involve food and eating.
- You ignore hunger signals by drinking extra amounts of water, tea, coffee, or diet sodas.
- You feel guilty when you eat something off your current diet plan.

- You use diet pills, caffeinated beverages, and cigarettes to reduce your appetite.
- You overexercise to compensate for perceived overeating or weight gain.
- You overuse laxatives and diuretics to combat overeating or bloating.
- You have excessive concern about your body size, which may include weighing yourself daily or multiple times per day.

Many clients I've worked with are or have been chronic dieters; and even if they're not currently dieting, they have difficulty giving up the diet mentality. While they know from experience with yo-yo weight loss and gain that diets don't work, they persist in thinking that if they just find the right diet, it will work *this* time. Hmm, magical thinking? I understand. I did the same thing for many years until I realized that *dieting was part of the problem.*

Chronic Low-Calorie Dieting Spells Trouble

Biochemistry researchers have proven without a shadow of doubt that chronic low-calorie dieting, interpreted by the body as starvation, harms our bodies and leads to overeating and weight gain.

The simple truth is that overly restrictive diets don't work, and they are not effective for long-term weight loss and maintenance. Chronic low-calorie dieting slows the metabolism. Your body, in its infinite wisdom, lowers its need for energy and becomes more efficient at utilizing calories. In addition, low-calorie dieting can trigger intense food cravings, and once we go off the diet, our bodies retain more fat in an attempt to store more energy before another famine arrives. Intense frustration, shame, guilt, and low self-esteem accompany weight gain and lead to the vicious cycle of searching for the next diet or trying one that you had some success with in the past.

Gaining weight is not the only consequence of low-calorie dieting. There are also serious health threats. Yo-yo dieters have an increased risk of heart disease and premature death, including sudden death syndrome.

Liquid fasting and diets of less than eight hundred calories per day can lead to gallstones and ultimate removal of the gallbladder. Low-calorie dieting can cause serious nutritional deficiencies and exhaust your adrenal glands, your first-response stress busters.

In order to reconnect to your signals, you must begin to release the diet mentality. This means eating when you feel true hunger, stopping when you're satiated, and allowing yourself a free choice of foods to satisfy your cravings.

Modern Foods Fool Our Machinery

Our calorie-counting machinery works best when we eat a diet consistent with our human design, a predominantly unprocessed, whole-foods, plant-based diet composed of fruits, vegetables, legumes, potatoes, whole grains, nuts, and seeds. This is the diet of our ancestors, who, over thousands of years, maintained their body weight in an optimum range. Our bodies get all the essential nutrients we need, including essential amino acids, essential fatty acids, carbohydrates, vitamins, and minerals, from such a diet.

The standard American diet differs from the diet of our ancestors in many significant ways. First, and of critical importance, our modern diets are deficient in plant foods full of fiber. Second, they are loaded with processed foods. And finally, our intake of animal-derived foods is excessive. Our bodies are unable to accurately measure caloric intake on this type of diet, and the result is that we can and do consume an excess of calories before our bodies register satiation. On the modern diet, we can no longer trust our signals to guide us.

Modern Drug-like Foods Are Addictive

We humans are hardwired to seek pleasure, avoid pain, and conserve energy. When it comes to food, we naturally gravitate toward easily available, pleasurable food and eat it until we've had enough. Foods loaded with calories tend to be more pleasurable. To most of us, a cheesy bacon burger and fries is more appealing than vegetable soup and salad; a hot fudge sundae is more appealing than a fruit salad. Just like Pavlov's dogs, we develop conditioned responses. Once we associate a particular food with pleasure, we are more apt to seek it out again.

Modern foods artificially concentrated with fat, sugar, and salt act like drugs and stimulate the release of powerful feel-good chemicals, known as endorphins, in the pleasure centers of the brain. They also stimulate the release of a chemical called dopamine, which drives us to seek more pleasure. Our bodies are wise — these chemicals have always been necessary for our survival as a species. They drive us to seek pleasure by eating the most calorie-dense foods we can find and engaging in pleasurable activities, like mating with an appealing partner.

According to David A. Kessler, MD, author of *The End of Overeating*, "Chronic exposure to highly palatable foods changes our brains, conditioning us to seek continued stimulation. Over time, a powerful drive for a combination of sugar, fat, and salt competes with our conscious capacity to say no." He terms the resulting behavior "conditioned hypereating." He suggests that this behavior involves a "high degree of sensitivity" (to these artificially concentrated foods), "a perceived loss of control, an inability to feel satisfied, and obsessive thinking." Sounds like addiction, doesn't it? In sensitive individuals, even the aroma or just a taste of a food can trigger this conditioned hypereating. And because these foods are highly pleasing and calming, stress and intense emotional states can overpower our best intentions, heighten the power of the food as a cue, and drive us to seek out these foods.

We can, however, without too much effort, withdraw from addictive foods. We can resensitize ourselves to whole, unprocessed foods in a short period, usually one to three months. Our taste buds will readapt, and our cravings for artificially concentrated foods will diminish.

Inherited Conditions Throw Off Our Signals

There are many genetic or inherited conditions that cause body and brain imbalances. Those of particular importance to overeaters include hormonal irregularities, low or high levels of brain chemicals, and food allergies and sensitivities.

Did you know that hormone irregularities can result in blood sugar fluctuations, food cravings, mood instability, fatigue, overeating, and weight gain? Our finely calibrated endocrine system is composed of organs that secrete these hormones, compounds that affect the function of other organs and tissues. A malfunction in any of these organs — which include the adrenals, thyroid, pancreas, ovaries, and testes — can lead to appetite, mood, and energy disturbances.

Brain chemicals regulate our mood, mental energy, alertness, focus, and calmness. Our brain chemicals can become too low or high from inherited conditions such as mood disorders and thyroid disease. In addition, factors such as stress, season changes, drug and alcohol use, poor diet, low-calorie dieting, bingeing, and purging wreak havoc on our brain chemicals. When our brain chemicals are imbalanced, we may experience strong cravings for modern drug-like foods or beverages in an attempt to regulate our brain chemistry — to reduce anxiety, lift depression, calm down, rev up, focus, numb out, or tranquilize. If you're "not a morning person," you've probably already discovered the energizing effect a strong cup of coffee or tea has on your brain chemicals.

Food allergies and sensitivities occur when our immune system misperceives something we ingest as foreign. Some reactions, such as rashes or hives, are strong and clear, and we are likely to avoid the offender. Other reactions, such as food cravings, fatigue, water retention, foggyheadedness, headaches, inflammation, and irritability are less easily associated with particular foods. Before we experience these unpleasant symptoms, we may initially feel good after ingesting allergenic substances. This is because they can initially trigger a release of those feelgood opiate-like brain chemicals. Over time we can become addicted to these pleasurable chemicals. And our health can suffer if our immune system, designed to wage war on things like viruses, bacteria, and cancer cells, is constantly overstimulated by allergens.

Hectic Lifestyles Erode Our Health

Our lives today are full of stress. We've grown accustomed to the stress from demanding jobs, financial pressures, work and family commitments, social and relationship challenges, traffic, noise, and environmental toxins. We consider it normal to work long hours, skip meals, grab junk food on the run, expose our bodies to toxic chemicals, use stimulants to keep going, and, in general, ignore bodily needs for exercise, rest, rejuvenation, and sleep.

While stress in small doses can at times be useful, our bodies are not designed for chronic stress. They are designed to handle acute stressors followed by longer periods of rest. We can handle the notice of a potential job layoff, but add to it an impending home foreclosure and we've reached our limit. Our adrenal glands begin to overproduce stress hormones, and as they become overtaxed, other hormonal systems become affected.

We pay a price for our 24/7 lifestyles: lack of exercise and sleep contribute to endocrine malfunction. Regular physical exercise and adequate sleep are not just for weight management; they are also important aspects of good health. Both physical activity and proper rest relieve stress by regulating hormones. Both improve the overall quality of our lives and reduce our risk for several health conditions and diseases.

You Can Tune Up Your Chemistry and End Overeating

The five principles of balanced biochemistry that follow will assist you in correcting the physical imbalances that lead to low brain and body energy, compulsive food cravings, overeating, and weight gain. Even if you've taken poor care of yourself for a prolonged period and need to make changes in many of these areas, you *will* be able to overcome your overeating. Don't lose faith. It's never too late to take charge of your health. Baby step by baby step, you'll be taking better care of yourself and feeling healthier and more motivated to continue in a higher-functioning body.

The Five Principles of Balanced Biochemistry

We began addressing emotional eating in part 1 by tuning in to the emotions, thoughts, and needs that drive our behavior and building the skills needed to take the best care of ourselves. But not all overeating or all consumption of comfort food is emotional — some of it is caused by body and brain imbalances.

If you want to put an end to overeating, you'll need to rely on properly functioning body and brain signals to guide you toward balance. These five principles will show you how to tune in to your body and brain messages and help you correct any physical imbalances. By the process of elimination you'll be able to see what part of your eating still results from underlying emotional, cognitive, or spiritual imbalances and address those as well. If addressing the physical imbalances resolves your overeating, you may be one of the lucky few who just needs a biochemical tune-up.

Principle #1. Pay attention to hunger and fullness signals.

Principle #2. Eat foods consistent with your human design: unprocessed, whole plant foods.

Principle #3. Address body and brain imbalances.

Principle #4. Move your body.

Principle #5. Sleep to satiation.

In this section of the book, you'll discover

- how to pay attention to your basic body signals such as hunger, cravings, and fullness;
- which foods are most consistent with your human design;
- how to make the transition to a more body-slimming, health-promoting fare;
- how to recognize various bodily symptoms as signals of imbalance caused by

    - hormonal irregularities,
    - low or high levels of brain chemicals, and
    - food allergies and sensitivities;

- how to address biochemistry imbalances;
- how stress affects your body and how to reduce it;
- the importance of moving your body; and
- the importance of getting enough sleep.

It will take time to put all the principles in this section of the book into practice. Some of the principles you can begin to practice immediately, while others will require you to first make lifestyle adjustments or work with a health care provider. If you feel stalled on any principle, you can always begin practicing the next principle and later go back.

Remember to be gentle with yourself as you make lifestyle adjustments. Lack of motivation or willingness is often a result of blocked emotional areas. Practicing the self-care skills outlined in part 1 will help you work through these areas of imbalance and unlock the keys to your resistance.

It can be helpful to practice these principles with other family members or friends. These principles are truly for everyone, not just overeaters. Anyone who wants to feel better and have more energy will benefit.

CHAPTER EIGHT

Principle #1. Pay Attention to Hunger and Fullness Signals

Years of chronic dieting have taught many overeaters to be afraid of their hunger. Something as basic as listening to the wisdom of our bodies and eating when we're hungry feels unsafe. We're not sure we can trust our body signals to guide us. Perhaps we will eat everything in sight and never stop. What if we never feel satisfied? Lack of emotional nourishment in our lives has led us to associate hunger with emptiness and unmet needs.

We definitely did not start out this way. Infants and small children intuitively eat when they're hungry and stop eating usually before they're full. The truth is we *can* relearn to listen to our bodies and trust them to guide us. In order to do this, we must once and for all give up the idea of overly restrictive dieting.

If you've been a chronic dieter, you've probably learned lots of creative ways to ignore or dull your hunger signals. Perhaps you skip meals; drink calorie-free beverages such as coffee, tea, and diet sodas throughout the day; chew sugar-free gum; or smoke cigarettes. Maybe you try to stay as busy as possible to tune out hunger signals. These tricks, which are all attempts to fool the body, disconnect you from your body's wisdom and do not work well for sustained weight loss.

Many chronic dieters don't remember what it feels like to be hungry many times per day. Some try to decide through their thoughts whether they "deserve" to eat. Others eat according to the clock, whether they're hungry or not. And many tune out hunger by cutting it off at the pass: they eat large meals and lots of snacks and rarely register hunger.

Our metabolism slows down when we ignore our hunger signals, and putting off eating often leads to ravenous overeating later in the day. When you're used to ignoring your hunger, you may not notice the early subtle signals and may register hunger only when it is extreme.

Hunger Is Your Best Friend

Don't be afraid of your hunger. Welcome it — it's a wonderful signal and sign that your body is working properly and the machine is revving. Every time you feel true physical hunger, it's time to eat!

Hunger is a complex mechanism involving both brain and body — nature's way of making sure we survive. It involves signals of discomfort and tension that alert us that our reserves are low, as well as cravings that guide us as to which foods to choose. Pleasing tastes and the pleasurable chemicals released during digestion ensure we will come back for more. Once we begin to eat, our hunger signal fades and the pleasure of eating is reduced as we near satiation.

The hunger drive is part of our overall calorie-balancing process, and in combination with signals of satiety, or fullness, it helps us maintain optimal weight. In other words, our bodies naturally and without much effort will signal us to balance our intake of calories with our caloric expenditure. You may notice you are hungrier on the days when you exercise than on the days when you are less physically active. Your body is so wise that it even plays catch-up by increasing hunger if you have been eating too little for a number of days, such as when you are too busy or are ill. All of a sudden you find that your hunger seems relentless. Most women also notice that they feel hungrier two weeks before their menstrual period. The body, in its infinite wisdom, increases hunger because it needs more calories to build the uterine lining. Your body does lots of behind-the-scenes calculations to accomplish many tasks and maintain your body weight.

An important step in balancing your physical chemistry and ending overeating is to get back to basics by paying attention to your hunger signals and eating only when you feel true physical hunger. Any of the following may represent hunger:

- Gurgling, growling, or rumbling stomach noises
- A feeling of weakness or light-headedness
- Faintness
- Difficulty concentrating
- Irritability
- Headache

Eat When You Are Hungry

The best way to respond to your hunger is to eat according to internal cues, as opposed to the clock or your schedule. Allow yourself to get acquainted with the unique way you experience hunger.

Choose a day when you can control your schedule to begin practicing paying attention to your hunger cues. Rather than thinking in terms of breakfast, lunch, and dinner, try to think in terms of refueling sessions. Whenever the tank is getting low, regardless of the time of day, it's time to "fill up." While most people feel hunger within an hour or two of being awake, some are not hungry until later. If you don't feel hunger until late morning, don't eat until then, even though it has been drilled into your head that you *must* eat an early breakfast. Wait until your body signals you. If you are hungry before bedtime, your body is letting you know that a light snack may be in order. Forget any rules you have heard regarding when to eat, and just pay attention to your hunger cues.

Charting Your Hunger

Check in with yourself throughout the day. Every time you want to eat, ask yourself the following questions:

"Am I hungry?"

"What physical symptoms am I experiencing?"

"What emotions, if any, am I experiencing?"
"What is my hunger level?"
"What am I hungry for?"

Use the Hunger/Fullness Scale and the Daily Eating Log as often as possible to help you become more aware of your hunger signals and emotions before and after eating. Try to eat when you are at level 3 or 4 on the scale. Waiting until level 0–2 may lead to ravenous overeating. Notice that your hunger signal will vary from day to day according to your activity level and bodily needs.

Write down anything you notice about your eating behavior, such as "I notice hunger only when I'm starving, and then I grab anything in sight," or, "I never allow myself to get very hungry — it doesn't feel safe."

Hunger/Fullness Scale	
0___1___2___3___4___5___6___7___8___9___10 Very hungry Satisfied Stuffed	
0	Extremely hungry, ravenous, empty feeling, dizzy, shaky, difficulty concentrating (too hungry, you risk overeating)
1—2	Very hungry, noisy stomach, irritable (you risk overeating)
3	Strong desire to eat, no strong physical symptoms (best time to begin eating)
4	Mildly hungry — a few bites of something would do
5	*Hunger is gone! Body needs are met!*
6	Past hunger satisfaction: you're eating more food than your body requires, wanting to eat a bit more for taste
7	Getting uncomfortable, bloated, and lethargic
8	Beyond full; feeling remorse
9	Very uncomfortable
10	Stuffed: holiday dinner–style eating

Daily Eating Log

DATE:

Time	Physical symptoms and emotions before eating	Hunger scale	Type of food	Fullness scale	Physical symptoms and emotions after eating
		0 1 2 3 4 5 6 7 8 9 10		0 1 2 3 4 5 6 7 8 9 10	
		0 1 2 3 4 5 6 7 8 9 10		0 1 2 3 4 5 6 7 8 9 10	
		0 1 2 3 4 5 6 7 8 9 10		0 1 2 3 4 5 6 7 8 9 10	
		0 1 2 3 4 5 6 7 8 9 10		0 1 2 3 4 5 6 7 8 9 10	
		0 1 2 3 4 5 6 7 8 9 10		0 1 2 3 4 5 6 7 8 9 10	
		0 1 2 3 4 5 6 7 8 9 10		0 1 2 3 4 5 6 7 8 9 10	

Things I noticed about my eating behavior today:

There Are No Forbidden Foods

When you experience true physical hunger, I want you to select whatever foods look good to you. I'm not going to tell you there is any food you can't eat. That would just trigger a sense of deprivation and a rebellion of your *feeling self.* If you want grains and fruit for breakfast, go for it. Perhaps you prefer lentil soup and a potato. If you want a slice of chocolate cake and ice cream, choose that. Yes, you read correctly. Allowing yourself a free choice of foods when you're hungry will lessen any sense of restriction you may feel. Eating foods you believe you *should* eat but don't want to eat only leads to feeling deprived. And there's a high probability that later you will overeat the foods that you really wanted. At this point in the program, I'm not concerned with *what* you eat; I just want you to eat *only* when you feel true physical hunger. As you become more balanced in mind, body, and spirit, you will naturally begin to make healthier choices.

Pay attention to your cravings. Cravings are part of the hunger drive, signaling you to eat foods that supply nutrients your body needs. When your body needs vitamin C, it will signal you with cravings for things like oranges and strawberries. When your body needs fat, then rich foods like avocados and nuts will look good. Cravings should go away soon after eating. If you have strong cravings for drug-like junk foods and you feel compelled to eat these foods, you may have an allergic addiction. I address food allergies in principle #3, in chapter 10. At this point, just note which foods trigger compulsiveness.

Your cravings may also be highlighting an emotional appetite. Many emotional eaters can't tell the difference between a true physical appetite and an emotional appetite. Often emotional hunger feels just like physical hunger. Let me suggest that if you're uncertain whether you're truly physically hungry, ask yourself the following question: Did I eat enough food throughout the day yesterday and today? If you did not, your hunger may be physical, even if you just ate a big meal. Your body may be signaling you that it did not get enough calories or nutrients recently. If it is already late in the day, then it's best to have a light snack, if possible, such as a piece of fruit, or some fruit with a few nuts, and begin fueling first thing in the morning. If you believe you did eat enough yesterday and today, and you have a strong desire to keep eating, try a light snack; if the hunger continues, it may very well be emotional. Focusing your efforts on the self-care skills in part 1 of this book will help you address your emotional hunger.

Please note that if you have been diagnosed with insulin resistance or diabetes, you will have to be mindful of your food intake, especially of foods that convert to sugar quickly. Having to watch your food intake carefully may intensify the feeling of deprivation and trigger emotional eating. I have found that the best way to work this program and *work with* these metabolic imbalances is to still allow forbidden foods periodically, but in limited quantities. Try to strike a balance — practice setting limits (skill #4, in chapter 5) and *consciously* allow yourself a few bites of a favorite forbidden food. Do this often enough that you don't feel deprived, but infrequent enough that it doesn't unbalance you too much. The key here is to *consciously choose* your forbidden foods rather than to sneak them or binge on them. Keep in mind that we all need to eat our favorite junk foods in moderation. You'll need to work closely with your health care practitioner before making any changes to your diet or medications.

"What If I Get Hungry and There Is No Food Around?"

"I wasn't hungry when I woke up, so I headed out to run errands. When I got hungry, I grabbed junk because I couldn't wait until I got home."

"Dinner with my husband got postponed an hour, and by the time we sat down to eat I was so hungry I devoured the bread basket."

Paying attention to your hunger signals also means anticipating your hunger and making sure you have food with you when you're away from home. You will need to get in the habit of carrying food with you. I generally carry things like fresh fruit, nuts, corn or rice cakes, a baked potato, rice and beans, and a bottle of water. I carry food in the car, and I keep some additional, nonperishable foods, like instant soup and oatmeal, in my office drawer. This way I never find myself hungry and without food I can eat.

Perhaps you resist the idea of carrying food with you because it seems bothersome and too much work. What you're really resisting is taking care of yourself. Just as a good parent packs a bag of food for a day out with a toddler, you must be a good parent to yourself. Making sure you have something to eat when you're hungry is a nurturing act.

"What If I Have a Lunch or Dinner Engagement and I'm Not Hungry?"

There may be times when you have a busy work or social schedule and you choose to eat before you actually feel hunger signals. Maybe you've been invited to dinner and a movie with friends at 5:30 PM, and you don't normally eat until 7 PM, or you ate a late lunch. This is a time when you may choose to go ahead and eat a small amount even though you have no noticeable hunger signals. You could also take some food with you and nibble on it during the movie.

"I Seem to Be Eating All the Time"

Responding to your hunger by eating mini meals many times per day keeps you satisfied and maintains energy better than larger meals. It is normal and natural to follow a grazing style, where you eat four to six small meals per day.

Many overeaters do not eat this often. Some with fast metabolisms tell me that it's too much effort to eat every time they are hungry, so they often eat larger, fattier meals to carry them for long periods. They prefer to "eat and be done with it." Your body is wise, and it reads this large meal as a signal: "Store for the coming famine!" It will rapidly store these excess fat calories as fat.

Those with slower metabolisms who experience milder hunger signals often go without food or eat very little during most of the day and then overeat at night. They pack in the calories when their bodies have slowed down for the day. They often tell me that once they start eating, they can't stop. This may be an indication that their appetite-stimulating and -suppressing hormones have become imbalanced because they regularly wait too long to eat and then overeat.

Both groups are throwing their signals off by eating too infrequently and eating too much at one sitting. Eating more often definitely means more food-gathering and preparation. This is one of the many ways we humans take care of ourselves. Our early ancestors spent *a lot* of time gathering and preparing food. Wild animals often spend *most* of their day searching for food. At least we need only spend part of our day gathering and preparing, and we don't have to roam the plains or at times go hungry!

"What If I Want to Eat and I'm Not Hungry?"

At some point you *will* want to eat when you're *not* hungry. That's why you're reading this book. You eat for a multitude of reasons, not all of them related to physical hunger. At these times, write down the emotions prompting you to want to use food for any other reasons. You may find you're desperately uncomfortable when you no longer make food your source of soothing and comfort. Perhaps you're unsure of what you're feeling other than a desire for pleasure and distraction. Maybe you *are* aware of unpleasant emotions surfacing but don't know what to do with them or how to comfort yourself. Be gentle and patient with yourself. You may still want to overeat and to numb these emotions, and that's okay. But before you do, try having an Inner Conversation (skill #1, in chapter 2). See if you can access your Inner Nurturer's voice and then comfort and soothe your *feeling self*. Even if you give in to the urge to overeat, you are well on your way to ending emotional eating. Consider it a success if you used the daily log, had an Inner Conversation, or just considered using these tools.

"It's Hard to Get Myself to Write Down What I Eat"

When you use the log, you will certainly feel more conscious of what you put in your mouth. You may feel resistant to focusing on your hunger and eating, however. Charting your hunger and fullness may remind you of past diets and deprivation. Do you fear that someone will find your log and judge your eating? Are *you* judging your eating? Do you feel as if writing it down will force you to be "good" and kill the joy of mindless eating?

Remind yourself that you are no longer going on overly restrictive diets. No more weighing or measuring food or counting calories. The log is not about dieting or being perfect with your food. It's just as legitimate to list chocolate on the log as it is blueberries. No judgment, just observations of habits and patterns. Take note of all the emotions surfacing and commit to using the log anyway.

You don't have to use the log for every snack or meal or even every day. If you notice you're feeling rebellious, write down what you're feeling and, if you need to, take a day off from using it. The log is merely a tool to help you tune in to your body's signals and take the best care of yourself.

When It's Time to Stop Eating

You've probably never heard of something Doug J. Lisle, PhD, and Alan Goldhamer, DC, authors of *The Pleasure Trap*, call the "stretch sensation," even though you've experienced it many times. We have nerves called stretch receptors embedded in our stomachs, which get stimulated once we start eating. They signal us as to how much our stomachs are being stretched by the food we eat. In addition to the stretch sensation, our bodies make complex calculations regarding the calories and nutrients of the foods we eat and the fullness of our body-fat reserves. Our phenomenal machines do all this calculating in an attempt to shut down our appetites and help us stop eating.

Fullness is an important biological signal designed to make sure we don't overeat, get fat and sluggish, and become easy food for a predator. Drs. Lisle and Goldhamer state that our satiation mechanisms are part of a universal law of nature that they call the Law of Satiation. The law states, "In a natural setting of caloric abundance, animals will consume the correct amount of food needed for optimal function." Animals in the wild are never overweight, because they eat according to this natural law. And this is why our early ancestors, even during times of abundance, were not overweight.

At some point after we have begun eating, generally within about twenty minutes, our stretch receptors will give us a subtle signal that we've had enough. It doesn't take a lot of food to trigger the stretch sensation; even a large apple can trigger it. If we ignore this signal, our stretch receptors will send a louder signal. If your tendency is to eat everything on your plate, you're probably eating beyond the first signal. You would end up eating half to three-quarters of most meals if you stopped at the first stretch sensation.

Charting Your Fullness

In order to stop eating when you first feel the stretch sensation, or soon after, you'll have to become more mindful of this signal. To learn to do so, it's best to eat alone and without distraction. If you're dining socially, you might want to excuse yourself and go to the restroom midmeal to check in with yourself.

Using the Hunger/Fullness Scale and Daily Eating Log, try to assess the level of fullness each time you eat. Take a brief break whenever you are eating and check in with your body. You should feel the initial subtle stretch sensation somewhere around level 5. Check your level of satisfaction at this point. Can you stop now and remind yourself there is no restriction? You get to eat again the minute your body gives you the hunger signal. Do you feel resistance to stopping at this point? Take a moment and ask yourself what emotions this might be bringing up. Jot these emotions down in your log. Try to stop eating somewhere between level 5 and level 6.

"What If I Can't Tell I'm Full Until I'm Really Full?"

If you notice only the louder fullness, or stuffed, signals, it's generally because you're eating too fast or your meals lack fiber. Our stretch receptors generally work well, and they work best when we eat slowly and consume foods with fiber. The standard American diet, which is often very low in fiber and high in animal-derived foods and processed foods, gives us an abundance of calories before we register the stretch sensation. You may not feel any stretch sensation from a cup of ice cream, but you *will* feel it from a large apple with peanut butter. You won't feel the stretch sensation from four small pieces of chocolate, but you *will* feel it from a small bag of carrot sticks plus hummus.

"I Feel Deprived When I Stop at the Stretch Sensation"

Allow yourself time to become acquainted with how the varying stages of fullness feel, from the first subtle signal to the feeling of being stuffed and almost ill. Notice your level of satisfaction at each stage. Not wanting to stop when your body signals "enough" is a sign that either you haven't been refueling often enough or you're eating for emotional reasons. If it's too challenging to stop at the stretch sensation, still try to stop eating at some point before your usual stopping place. If you regularly eat until stuffed, try stopping a few bites before you're stuffed. If you often eat to a comfortable full feeling, try stopping a few bites before you're full. Even though you may choose to eat beyond the early subtle stretch sensation, can you eat slowly enough to feel the first cue?

Stopping at the stretch sensation will most likely mean leaving appealing food on your plate. If you're dining out, you may have not yet tried all the delectable foods on the table. If you take the food home, it's true that it won't be as fresh and delicious tomorrow. Stay mindful of your goal to pay attention to your fullness signals. Remind yourself that you've had enough food for now and that there will be many more opportunities to eat incredibly tasty food.

Take note of your energy after you eat. Do you feel energized and ready for your next activity? Do you feel sleepy, sluggish, and ready for a nap? This will give you clues about how the foods you are choosing affect you and how much is the right amount.

Remember, you are not restricted; you can eat as much as you like, and there are no forbidden foods. At this point, the goal is to pay attention to your hunger and fullness signals, to begin eating when you are hungry, and to stop eating at some point before you are very full.

"I Feel Guilty Leaving Food on My Plate"

Many of us were raised to "clean our plates" because, as we were told, somewhere in the world there are starving children. The problem with this outdated philosophy is that it encourages us to eat according to the amount of food on the plate rather than according to our body signals. And, of course, finishing the last portion on the plate, or polishing off the whole bag of cookies, does nothing for those starving children; it only adds to *our* hip and waist sizes. Sometimes, when taking food home or eating it as leftovers is not an option, a little waste is inevitable.

In America, we are used to preparing large portions, and restaurants too tend to serve huge amounts. When we're not fully conscious of our eating, it's easy to eat until we're stuffed. As you get better acquainted with your body signals, you'll be better able to gauge how much food to prepare or order. At restaurants, it might be best to share meals or have the waiter wrap up half your meal from the start. This is a great way to ensure that you will stop before you're full. It's also a good idea to push the food away from you once you feel full.

"How Can I Pay Attention to My Signals at Parties?"

Social functions and parties can lead to trouble — the combination of social distraction and an overabundance of rich, processed food can result in unconscious eating. Even at social gatherings, we can tune in to our body signals and stop eating when we get the appropriate signal. If you had a child with you, you would, as a good parent or guardian, tune in to what the child was eating. This is what you must practice doing with yourself. This doesn't have to mean deprivation. You can still sample many of the delectable foods you have your eye on — your signals will guide you when to stop. Try practicing my three social eating rules.

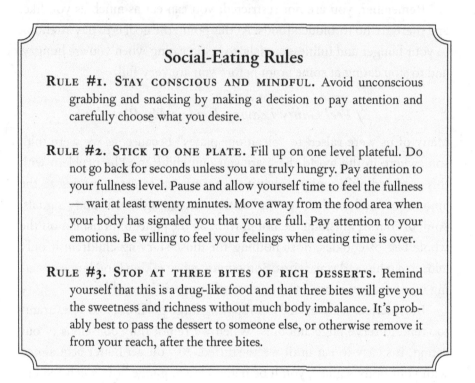

Social-Eating Rules

RULE #1. STAY CONSCIOUS AND MINDFUL. Avoid unconscious grabbing and snacking by making a decision to pay attention and carefully choose what you desire.

RULE #2. STICK TO ONE PLATE. Fill up on one level plateful. Do not go back for seconds unless you are truly hungry. Pay attention to your fullness level. Pause and allow yourself time to feel the fullness — wait at least twenty minutes. Move away from the food area when your body has signaled you that you are full. Pay attention to your emotions. Be willing to feel your feelings when eating time is over.

RULE #3. STOP AT THREE BITES OF RICH DESSERTS. Remind yourself that this is a drug-like food and that three bites will give you the sweetness and richness without much body imbalance. It's probably best to pass the dessert to someone else, or otherwise remove it from your reach, after the three bites.

Occasionally eating beyond fullness at social functions does not have to derail you or ruin all your good progress. As long as you don't do this at every refueling session, you'll be fine.

Don't Forget to Hydrate Your Body

Thirst, like hunger and fullness, is a powerful biological signal, and it drives us to seek water. Drinking adequate amounts of water throughout the day allows us to stay well hydrated and keeps our signals functioning properly. By the time we become thirsty, we are already slightly dehydrated — our thirst signal is informing us that we now have a window of time in which to safely rehydrate.

Symptoms of mild to moderate dehydration may include the following:

- Headache
- Dizziness or light-headedness
- Muscle weakness
- Sleepiness or fatigue
- Dry mouth
- Decreased urine output

If your urine is colorless or pale yellow, consider yourself well hydrated. Dark yellow urine usually signals dehydration, unless it's the result of taking B vitamins, which make it bright amber or bright yellow.

How Much Water Should You Drink?

The Institute of Medicine, an independent, nonprofit, nongovernmental American organization that provides unbiased and authoritative advice to decision makers and the public, suggests we let thirst be our guide. They advise women to consume about 9 cups (2.2 liters) of total beverages a day, and men to consume roughly 13 cups (3 liters). On average, food provides about 20 percent of total water intake — many fruits and vegetables are 90–100 percent water by weight. You'll need to get the remaining 80 percent from pure water and other beverages. Juice and noncaffeinated herbal teas can contribute but should not constitute the majority of your fluid intake.

It's best to drink fluids out of reusable glass containers. Avoid plastic containers that can leach toxic chemical residues and cause hormonal imbalance. And, of course, less plastic means we help avoid overwhelming our recycling capacities.

CHAPTER NINE

Principle #2. Eat Foods Consistent with Your Human Design: Unprocessed, Whole Plant Foods

If you have struggled with emotional eating and have been overweight for a long time, you have probably already tried many diets, perhaps even with some success. But you may be unclear about how to lose the weight and keep it off without constantly feeling hungry and deprived. Decades of the cultural diet-mentality and the overconsumption of calorie-rich processed foods and foods of animal origin have disconnected many of us from our intuitive body wisdom.

There is always much debate surrounding the issue of diet. You may be left wondering: Which is the *correct* eating plan? Are carbohydrates okay to eat, or should I limit them? Should I follow a high-protein or low-to-moderate-protein eating plan? How much fat should I eat, and what types? Is it healthy to eat animal products, including dairy and eggs, or should I cut them out and follow a plant-based eating plan?

There is one thing that most of the experts agree on: our modern diet is a far cry from the plant-based, unprocessed, whole-foods diet that our ancestors ate. Long ago, we began to grill, bake, smoke, fry, and salt meats; pasteurize dairy products; and refine grains and fruits into denatured, fiberless flour and sugar products. We've created things like refined vegetable oils, trans fats, and high-fructose corn syrup. We've canned and packaged food and added toxic ingredients like dyes and preservatives.

Over time, the human diet has been slowly increasing in animal products, highly refined processed foods, and foods artificially concentrated in proteins, fats, and sugars and deficient in plant fiber. You never see foods with these concentrations of protein, fat, and sugar in nature.

We are consuming less plant food than ever before in our history. Our nomadic ancestors were constantly on the move, and they ate a lot of wild plant foods full of fiber. We can maintain our best health and optimum weight by consuming at least thirty grams of fiber each day. Fiber helps to fill you up and turn off your appetite. Did you know that plant-eating animals that are our size in nature eat thirty to ninety grams or more of fiber per day? Plant foods provide our bodies with all the essential nutrients needed — amino acids, essential fatty acids, complex carbohydrates, phytochemicals, vitamins, and minerals. Our body chemistry and biochemical signaling system get thrown off when we consume a low-fiber diet filled with animal products and processed foods.

A key component of the hunger drive is the tendency to prefer the most calorically dense foods available. This means our bodies signal us to choose foods with a lot of calories in order to sustain life. Plant fiber increases the amount of stretch-receptor activity (discussed in chapter 8) in our digestive tract and helps our machinery get an accurate calorie count. So what are we going to do when we're regularly bombarded with an overabundance of high-calorie, fiber-deficient animal products and processed foods? We're going to feel powerfully driven to eat these foods all the time until satiated. The flaw is not in our human design. The problem is the standard American diet.

We all know that substances like sugar, alcohol, caffeine, and tobacco can lead to addiction in sensitive individuals. But did you know that calorically dense foods, especially fatty meats and dairy products (like ribs, franks, burgers, and cheese), processed foods containing fats and refined sugars (like ice cream and milk chocolate), and highly refined (non-whole-) grain products (like scones, bagels, pretzels, crackers, and many cereals) act like drugs and trigger the release of pleasurable chemicals in our brains? They do, and we can easily become addicted to them. And once we experience this intense pleasure from dense-calorie animal products and processed foods, we experience them as more pleasurable than whole-plant foods, making the reintroduction and transition to whole foods a bit more challenging.

Our dietary excesses and convenience-focused lifestyles have led to — in addition to food addiction — the diseases of excess. These include heart disease, stroke, diabetes, hypertension, diverticulitis, gall and kidney stones, osteoporosis, arthritis, gout, cancer, tooth decay, and obesity.

I want to introduce you to an eating plan that is sustainable — one that will be satisfying and satiating and that will both maintain your ideal weight and maximize your health and energy.

On a plant-based, unprocessed-whole-foods eating plan, your body chemistry becomes balanced and your biochemical signals (hunger, cravings, and fullness) work well. Each time you eat, you feel satisfied and balanced physically and emotionally. You'll feel mentally focused and physically energized for a few hours after each meal. If you love to eat, you may still think about food often, but you'll be free of compulsive cravings driven by imbalanced biochemistry.

On this eating plan, all your needs for protein, calcium, and other important nutrients can be met if you eat enough calories each day from a wide variety of unprocessed, whole plant foods. Whole foods have just the right balance of nutrients that our bodies require. Nature is wise. While your diet will be predominantly carbohydrates (the main fuel your body and brain use), all the foods you'll be eating will have protein, carbohydrates, and some fat. The only nutrient you may not get from your diet and may need to supplement with is vitamin B_{12}, which is not present in plants or meat, as it is made by bacteria. However, many vegetarian foods, including miso and soy milk, are fortified with this nutrient, so it is not difficult to get the recommended amount.

What Does a Plant-Based, Unprocessed-Whole-Foods Eating Plan Consist Of?

Our body signals work best when we eat foods consistent with our human design. When we eat whole plant foods, we work *with* our body rather than against it. We can trust our intuitive body wisdom to tell us when to eat, to select the right foods, and to signal us to stop eating when we've had enough. We can eat as much as we like and still lose weight effortlessly, without feeling hungry.

Fresh vegetables, fresh fruits, legumes (beans and lentils), potatoes, whole grains, nuts, and seeds are the foundation of vibrant health. This is essentially the diet we humans have been eating for millennia.

When many people hear "whole foods" or "plant-based eating plans," they think raw sprouts, fruits, veggies, and sparse eating plans that not only would be boring but also would take all the pleasure out of eating. This couldn't be further from the truth. This eating plan includes many foods you are already consuming. Many Indian, Thai, Chinese, Mexican, and even Italian meals you enjoy eating are predominantly plant based. You just need exposure to both cooked and raw plant foods and to their preparation to see for yourself that there will be plenty of pleasure left in dining.

Let me suggest that you remain open-minded as you read and explore this chapter. We all can become attached to things that give us pleasure, and food may be the only consistent source of pleasure in your life at this time. It's not always easy to change habits that were many years in the making. In fact, the mere suggestion of reducing your consumption of animal products and processed foods may make you want to put this book down and grab a dish of ice cream!

But before you exit this chapter because you think I'm going to try to convert you into a vegetarian or vegan overnight, let me share some thoughts with you. I'm not going to try to *take away* your favorite foods. My approach, always in baby steps, is to start by encouraging you to slowly *add* more unprocessed, whole plant foods to your diet. You can transition to this eating plan with just small, weekly changes. As you begin to *add* more wholesome foods to your diet, your palate and chemistry will change. Releasing foods that no longer serve your body becomes easy and effortless. Before discussing the specifics of the plan, let's look at some of the scientific rationale behind these healthful food choices.

Five Categories of Natural Whole Foods

VEGETABLES: Lettuce, spinach, chard, kale, collard greens, broccoli, cauliflower, cabbage, brussels sprouts, jicama, beets, celery, asparagus, artichokes, okra, leeks, mushrooms, radishes, carrots, onions, turnips, basil, cilantro, parsley, rhubarb, seaweed, butternut and acorn squash, pumpkin, zucchini, crookneck squash, eggplant, bell peppers, cucumbers, and tomatoes

FRUITS: Apples, bananas, oranges, grapefruits, tangerines, pears, apricots, melons, cherries, berries, peaches, nectarines, plums, grapes, pineapples, mangoes, kiwis, pomegranates, limes, lemons, raisins, dates, figs, prunes, avocados, and olives

LEGUMES AND POTATOES: Beans (adzuki, green, black, pinto, kidney, garbanzo, white, lima, fava, and others), soybeans, red and green lentils, black-eyed peas, dried split peas, fresh or frozen peas, snow peas, peanuts, and foods made from beans (hummus, refried beans, bean dips, miso, soy milk and soy yogurt, tofu, and tempeh); white, yellow, purple, and red potatoes, yams, and sweet potatoes

WHOLE GRAINS: wheat (bulghur and berries), spelt, buckwheat, oats, corn, brown rice, wild rice, barley, millet, rye, amaranth, sorghum, and quinoa

NUTS AND SEEDS: Almonds, walnuts, cashews, pistachios, pine nuts, Brazil nuts, macadamias, pecans, hazelnuts, coconuts, sunflower seeds, poppy seeds, sesame seeds, hemp seeds, pumpkin seeds, flaxseeds, and nut and seed butters

Carbohydrates Equal Satisfaction

The greatest need your body has is for fuel, and carbohydrates are your body's primary source. Your brain and nervous system rely exclusively on them. Your body is specially designed to process carbohydrates. At the tip of your tongue are taste buds that register sweetness, to encourage you to select the sweet tastes found in nature's complex and simple carbohydrates. Complex carbohydrates are starches like beans, grains, potatoes, and vegetables. Simple carbohydrates are found in fruits and in sweeteners such as agave nectar and maple syrup.

Once complex carbohydrates are in your mouth, your saliva, which contains the digestive enzyme alpha-amylase, begins to break them down into simple ones that can be more easily absorbed in your digestive tract.

Your twenty-six-foot-long tract is designed to efficiently handle large amounts of carbohydrates. Your body's capacity to store carbohydrates in your liver and muscles is, however, limited, so your body must constantly signal you, via cravings, to obtain a renewed supply. If your diet is deficient in carbohydrates, you may still be hungry even if you're feeling full.

If your diet is lacking in carbohydrates, your body will have to find other ways to supply energy. The body can convert protein, mainly from muscle tissue, to carbohydrates, but this is an expensive source of fuel. Protein is needed in the body to build, maintain, and repair things like muscles, hormones, and enzymes. Using your protein stores for fuel is like breaking down the walls of your home to build a nice fire in the fireplace. It will work, but at the cost of your structure — your muscle tissue. And don't be fooled into thinking that your body will start burning fat for energy if needed — only a small percentage of stored fat can be converted to carbohydrates and used as fuel. This process, called ketosis, occurs after a prolonged period of carbohydrate restriction or fasting, and the body *still* burns protein sources during ketosis.

Did you know that carbohydrates are the cleanest-burning fuel your body can use? Carbohydrates' main by-products are water and carbon dioxide, both of which can easily be eliminated from the body. In contrast, protein digestion results in the by-product nitrogen, which converts to urea and ammonia. Both of these can be harmful in large quantities, especially to the kidneys and liver.

The benefits of consuming wholesome, unprocessed, carbohydrate-rich foods extend well beyond physical health. Various studies by researchers at the Massachusetts Institute of Technology and elsewhere over the past twenty years have demonstrated that low-fat foods rich in carbohydrates boost the level of the brain chemical serotonin. This brain chemical not only improves mood and relieves depression but also helps control appetite and reduces bingeing. Foods rich in protein tend to reduce the level of serotonin.

Your hunger satisfaction, energy level, and good mood all rely on your consuming an adequate supply of carbohydrates. A plant-based whole-foods eating plan will easily meet your body's need for carbohydrates.

The Protein Hype

As Americans, we're always concerned with how much protein we're consuming, and we tend to think "more is better." According to the U.S. Food and Nutrition Board, the recommended dietary allowance of protein for the average adult is 0.8 grams per kilogram (2.2 pounds) of body weight. This amount, which includes a large margin of safety, translates into roughly 10 to 20 percent of your total daily calories. Human breast milk, *designed to support a growing infant*, is only 5 to 8 percent protein, and most of the calories are from carbohydrates. In the typical Western diet, the average American consumes roughly double the protein her body needs.

Highly popularized high-protein, low-carb diets such as the Atkins Diet or the South Beach Diet have scared a nation away from healthy, wholesome, unprocessed carbohydrates. Yet common sense tells you that any diet that shuns fresh fruit or starchy vegetables and encourages bacon, cheeseburgers, and cholesterol-lowering drugs can't be on the right track to vibrant health, optimum energy, and sustained weight loss. And while protein is a critical nutrient, too much of it can be just as bad as too much sugar, refined carbohydrates, or fat.

On severely carbohydrate-restricted, high-protein diets, people lose weight for three main reasons: first, they stop eating all the unhealthy processed carbohydrates (and therefore calories) they were eating; second, they lose water weight; and third, their bodies have to expend more calories to break down muscle tissue for fuel. Unfortunately, as demonstrated by many research studies, the weight lost generally doesn't stay off.

A study published in 2004 in the British medical journal the *Lancet* concluded that any weight loss advantage that Atkins and other low-carb diets may have is gone within a year. While there is better weight loss on these low-carb diets after six months, there is no difference after twelve months. In 2005, the *Journal of the American Medical Association* published the results of a comparison of four popular diets, including both the Atkins and Dr. Dean Ornish's low-fat, plant-based diet. At the one-year mark, those following the Ornish program had the greatest weight loss, while those following the Atkins program had the least weight loss.

The American Cancer Society conducted a study over a ten-year period with nearly eighty thousand participants who wanted to lose weight. Study participants who ate meat three times a week or more gained substantially more weight than those who avoided meat and ate more vegetables.

When we ingest protein, the acids and enzymes in the stomach begin to break it down into smaller compounds, called amino acids. Some of these amino acids are immediately used to repair and build muscle, hormones, skin, and other tissues. Since the body doesn't store protein and will not convert it to carbohydrates if there is sufficient carbohydrate intake for fuel, any excess protein has to be gotten rid of. Our kidneys, liver, and colon, unlike those of carnivorous animals, are ill-equipped to handle large amounts of animal proteins. These foods lack fiber and have significant amounts of fat and cholesterol. Carnivores have short intestines, which rotting, decomposing animal flesh quickly passes through. Protein digestion is a taxing process, and carnivorous animals sleep many hours of the day. Ever notice how many hours your dog or cat sleeps? Ever notice how sleepy you feel after a large meal rich in animal protein?

Excess protein is disposed of via your liver and kidneys and can result in the toxic buildup of harmful nitrogen-containing by-products. Diabetics and others already at a high risk of kidney disease increase this risk by consuming a high-protein diet. In addition, animal proteins are full of very acidic amino acids, known as sulfur-containing amino acids. Consuming a diet focused on meat, seafood, poultry, eggs, and dairy results in a high intake of acid many times per day. The body has to "rob" its bones, a great source of calcium, to buffer or neutralize all this acid. Calcium is also lost from the kidneys in large amounts when they must eliminate excess protein, especially animal protein. This increases the risk of developing painful kidney stones and diseases such as osteopenia and osteoporosis, in which the bones become overly porous. You can preserve your bones and actually reverse bone loss by consuming alkaline foods. Most fruits and vegetables are alkaline; and while most legumes and grains are acidic, they are far less acidic than animal proteins.

The consumption of animal proteins also plays a role in increasing your risk for cancer. Certain proteins present in meat, poultry, and fish when they are cooked at high temperatures (as in grilling and frying) have been found to produce compounds called heterocyclic amines. These substances have been linked to various cancers, including those of the breast and the colon.

High-protein diets that include the consumption of meat, eggs, and dairy products, all high in cholesterol, fat, and saturated fat, can increase your risk of heart disease. The most popular of these diets contain excessive amounts of these artery-clogging products. A plant-based, whole-foods eating plan is cholesterol-free and contains only small amounts of fat.

If we eat enough calories, we can get all the protein we need on a plant-based, whole-foods eating plan without injuring our bodies in the process. The best source of plant protein is the legume group, which includes beans, peas, and lentils. Also included in this group are soybeans and a variety of products made from soy, such as tofu, tempeh, and miso. Legumes are high-protein foods rich in calcium, iron, good fiber, and traces of essential fats. And they are easy to keep on hand — dried, frozen, or canned — to add to salads or soups. The U.S. government's National Health and Nutrition Examination Survey, conducted from 1999 through 2002, showed that people who included beans in their regular menu weighed, on average, six and a half pounds less than those who generally neglected this food group.

But don't worry — even if you hate beans, have trouble digesting them, or are allergic to them, you'll still get plenty of protein on a plant-based diet. Your body knows how to use the essential amino acids from foods like potatoes, yams, starchy winter squashes, corn, peas, brown rice, oats, barley, quinoa, and even broccoli and kale for building and repair functions. As my dear friend Dr. Janice Stanger, author of *The Perfect Formula Diet*, states, "You can target plant sources to get your essential amino acids and skip the animal middleman. No matter how much meat you eat, you manufacture your cells 100% from plant-formed or bacteria-formed amino acids. Animal protein is recycled plant protein."

Many clients have told me they tried a plant-based eating plan at some point in their lives and found they just did not feel well. They felt better when they went back to eating foods of animal origin. They erroneously concluded that all bodies are different and that some "need" animal proteins. They were resistant to trying a plant-based eating plan again.

I felt the same way. While I always believed that our original diet was predominantly plant based, and I felt guilty eating animals (and, in that way, participating in the slaughter of innocent sentient beings), every time I switched to a plant-based eating plan I felt worse. When I decided to try again, I consulted the writings of some of my favorite medical doctors who recommend a plant-based diet, and it became clear that I had never followed a truly *wholesome* plan. Previously, I had been more of a junky vegetarian, eating lots of processed foods and often not eating enough wholesome fruits, vegetables, legumes, potatoes, grains, nuts, and seeds. When I made the switch again, I felt much better and had lots of energy, and my cravings for sugar (I have always had a sweet tooth) dropped to near zero. I knew this was a way of eating I could sustain for life. So before you conclude that this eating plan isn't for you, make sure you're eating mostly whole, unprocessed foods.

The Skinny on Fats

The low-fat, no-fat mania of the 1990s led many Americans to steer clear of foods with fat. Yet contrary to popular opinion, *fat is an essential nutrient*. It's a component of every cell membrane in your body. Fat deposited under the skin helps to insulate your body and prevent rapid loss of heat. Fats cushion and support body organs like your brain and eyes, help make hormones, add luster to your hair, act as a backup energy supply, and help metabolize the fat-soluble vitamins A, D, E, and K.

Fatty foods are the most concentrated sources of calories, providing nine calories per gram (carbohydrates and protein provide only four calories per gram). Even though fatty foods are calorically dense, they don't provide a lot of energy. It's easier for your body to store fats than to burn them as fuel — remember, your body will burn available carbohydrates before it turns to protein or fat stores. Since most of the fat you eat is being stored, it's easy to add a pound of fat to your hips, thighs, rear end, or abdomen in a short amount of time just by consuming meals full of animal products and processed foods. And as you may have noticed, exercise alone won't get rid of the fat.

Fats can be broken down into "nonessential" and "essential" fats. While your body can synthesize the nonessential fats on its own, essential fats are substances your body cannot make and that you must obtain from your diet. Essential fats are made only by plants.

While wild animals and fish get their essential fatty acids directly from plant sources, the main sources of fatty acids for most Americans are meats, poultry, fish, and dairy products (we're basically eating animal products to get the essential fatty acids stored in their tissues), as well as vegetable oils and processed foods. Why not go directly to the source, the plants?

There are two essential fatty acids: alpha-linolenic acid and its derivatives (EPA and DHA), which are called the omega-3s; and linoleic acid and its derivatives (GLA, DGLA, and AA), which are called the omega-6s. The harder-to-get omega-3s are found in high concentrations in flaxseeds, hemp seeds, walnuts, pumpkin seeds, soybeans, kidney beans, and some coldwater fish. The omega-6s, which tend to be easily available and overconsumed in the standard American diet, can be found in processed foods containing hydrogenated fats and refined vegetable oils and animal products, including eggs, organ meats, cream, and butter. If you're eating a diet with a high concentration of animal products and processed foods, you may be consuming much higher levels of omega-6s than omega-3s. Research suggests that maintaining an optimal ratio of omega-6s to omega-3s is a key component of good overall health. While the optimal dietary ratio is still being debated, the consensus among nutritionists is that a ratio of no more than four to one is best. When you don't get enough of these essential fats, or when they're imbalanced, you can suffer from things like dry, scaly skin, breaking nails, hormonal havoc, mood disturbances, and food cravings.

Consuming a diet of unprocessed, wholesome plant foods is the best way to meet your need for essential fat. Two level tablespoons a day of ground flaxseed sprinkled on your favorite cereal, salad, soup, or smoothie will ensure that you're getting your omega-3s. Grind only enough for a few days and store the ground seeds in a tightly closed container in a cool, dry place. Once grinding has broken down the seeds' protective shell, the seeds begin to oxidize and lose their healthful qualities. Don't worry about getting enough omega-6s; you'll get plenty of them on this eating plan.

It's best to reduce or eliminate your intake of oils. Processed, extracted oils like vegetable, seed, and fruit oils are not found in nature. The process of extracting the oil discards all the other ingredients, such as fiber, protein, carbohydrates, vitamins, and minerals, from the whole food, creating an all-fat nonfood. Olive oil, for example, is actually a nonfood, even though we are told it's healthy. It would be better to eat the olive with all its fiber and nutrients. And when heated, many oils used for cooking break down into compounds called free radicals that can be harmful if consumed in large amounts.

Cow's Milk Is for Baby Cows

Did you know that there is no animal in nature that drinks the milk of another animal? We've been duped! The dairy industry has spent millions of dollars to convince you, your doctors, and your government agencies that you *need* cow's milk. We've grown up being told that we need to drink milk to build strong bones — that we need milk for calcium. This couldn't be further from the truth.

Numerous studies, including the Harvard Nurses' Health Study, which followed more than seventy-five thousand women for twelve years, have found no protective effect of dairy calcium on fracture risk or on bones. Researchers at Yale University found that the countries with the highest rates of osteoporosis — including the United States, Finland, and Sweden — were those in which people consumed the most milk, meat, and other animal products.

Dairy products, which include milk, butter, yogurt, ice cream, and cheese, contribute significant amounts of saturated fat and cholesterol to the diet. Diets high in fat and saturated fat can increase the risk of several chronic conditions, including obesity, heart disease, and diabetes.

Breast, prostate, and ovarian cancers have also been linked to the consumption of dairy products. The sugar in milk, lactose, is broken down in the body into another sugar, galactose. According to a study by Daniel Cramer, MD, and his colleagues at Harvard, some women have particularly low levels of the enzymes needed to break down galactose. When these women consume dairy products on a regular basis, their risk of ovarian cancer can be triple that of other women.

Many health challenges, including gastrointestinal distress, irritable bowel syndrome, diarrhea, and allergies, can be traced to the ingestion of dairy products. Lactose intolerance affects approximately 95 percent of Asian Americans, 74 percent of Native Americans, 70 percent of African Americans, 53 percent of Mexican Americans, and 15 percent of Caucasians.

The bottom line? Steer clear of dairy products. Nature never intended for you to drink another animal's milk. Soy, rice, oat, and low-fat nut or seed milks make good substitutes. A plant-based, whole-foods eating plan that eliminates dairy products and includes calcium-rich vegetables, such as leafy greens (like kale, collard, broccoli, and mustard greens), beans, and fortified grains, and juices will provide all the calcium your body requires.

The Evidence Is Mounting

The world's most important health advisory bodies have come to the same basic conclusion: the proper diet for humans is one that is plant-based and consists predominantly of whole foods. Consider the following:

- In 1991, the World Health Organization put out a detailed report stating that diets associated with increases in chronic diseases are those rich in sugar, meat and other animal products, saturated fat, and dietary cholesterol. The 2003 updated version took the same overall view as the previous report.

- In 1995, the Physicians Committee for Responsible Medicine issued a report urging the U.S. government to recommend a vegetarian diet to U.S. citizens. The committee's report stated, "The scientific literature clearly supports the use of vegetables, fruits, legumes (peas, beans, chick peas — pulses) and grains as staples. Meat, dairy products and added vegetable oils should be considered optional." The following year, the Dietary Guidelines for Americans promoted vegetarian diets for the first time.

- In 1997, the American Institute for Cancer Research issued a report, *Food, Nutrition, and the Prevention of Cancer: A Global Perspective*. The report recommended choosing a diet predominantly plant based, rich in a variety of vegetables, fruits, and legumes, with minimally processed starchy staple foods.

- And finally, in 2003, the American Dietetic Association and the Dietitians of Canada were firmly on board with meat-free diets, stating that heart disease, strokes, some cancers, and diabetes can all be effectively treated by prescribing a vegetarian diet.

The Benefits Extend beyond Improved Health and Weight Loss

I realize that just knowing that an eating plan is better for your health doesn't always translate into a change in eating habits. For sure, it's difficult to let go of foods we've grown attached to, especially those that give us comfort, even though we know they aren't good for us. Let me share with you some additional benefits you'll experience that may encourage you to make the shift.

You can eat until you're full. *How much* you eat is much less important than *what* you eat.

You can have snacks whenever you want them. You can choose to eat three meals and a few snacks, or eat mini meals every few hours.

There is a tremendous variety of foods to choose from. Nature's garden is bursting with interesting tastes, flavors, and aromas. There is no reason to be bored on this plan.

You'll be eating lots of satisfying carbohydrates, including starchy foods like corn on the cob, potatoes, beans, lentils, and wholesome grains like brown rice and barley.

You'll have regular bowel movements, woo hoo, eliminating lots of toxic waste!

You'll have fewer out-of-balance food cravings, or none at all.

You'll eliminate the fear and shame you may have been harboring regarding degenerative conditions such as diabetes, hypertension, and heart disease.

You'll reduce the amount of inflammation in your body. Eliminating animal products and processed foods translates into fewer inflammatory ailments, including headaches, stomachaches, sinus problems, and joint pains.

You will strengthen your immune system, which means fewer colds, less flu, and better health in general. When your body's first line of defense isn't tied up fighting off foreign proteins and allergens, it is free to go after viruses, bacteria, and wayward cancer cells.

Your skin will look better. A multinational study found that while wholesome plant foods protect your skin, meat, dairy, butter, margarine, and sugar were associated with increased skin damage.

You'll have more energy, better sleep, and overall improved health.

You'll save money on food and health care costs.

You'll be saving the lives of many sentient farm animals. Billions of animals are slaughtered each year in America for human consumption. They live short lives full of trauma and suffering. When you stop eating animal products, you say no to this unnecessary cruelty.

And you'll be treading more lightly on the earth and reducing your ecological footprint. By reducing your demand for animal products, you help stop the air pollution from manure and farmed animal transport, reduce the use of pesticides and herbicides used to grow animal feed, and prevent further depletion of fish populations and destruction of marine habitats. All win-win!

Making the Transition

You can begin your transition to a whole-foods eating plan by adding more plant foods to your diet each week. Keep in mind that you do not have to make this shift overnight. You can make it slowly and gradually. Taking time to make the transition reduces resistance and any sense of deprivation. Since you may be trying and preparing new foods, it will take time to figure out what to buy, where to buy it, and how to prepare it. Allow yourself the time you need for this process.

As you add more plant foods each week, your biochemistry will change and your preferences and cravings will begin to shift. You may want to release certain foods because they simply do not appeal to you anymore. You may find that stopping consumption of animal products completely is the easiest way. Or you may choose to keep a small amount of animal products in your diet. This is a personal choice.

If you feel you will not or cannot give up animal products, fear not. There is still hope for you. This program is for vegans, vegetarians, and meat eaters alike. I will not tell you there is any food you cannot eat. That would just lead to a rebellion by your *feeling self* and to food sneaking or bingeing. Just remember that the less you eat of animal products (including fish, dairy, and eggs), processed foods, sugars, and oils, the better your body will work. This translates into fewer cravings, easier weight loss, and better health.

Eight Simple Steps

You can make the transition to this eating plan in eight easy steps. Most of my recommendations for servings per day are based on the guidelines set by the Physicians Committee for Responsible Medicine. Whenever possible, choose organic foods over those that are conventionally grown with pesticides.

1. Increase Your Intake of Vegetables

In particular, eat plenty of dark yellow and orange starchy vegetables, like carrots, squash, corn, and pumpkin; and dark green leafy vegetables, like broccoli, kale, chard, collards, and mustard greens. Try building a meal around starchy vegetables such as corn and winter squash. Vegetables are good sources of fiber and are packed with nutrients such as beta-carotene, vitamin C, riboflavin, calcium, and iron. *Aim for three or more servings per day.* SERVING SIZE: one cup of raw vegetables; one-half cup of cooked vegetables.

2. Increase Your Intake of Legumes (Beans, Peas, and Lentils) and Potatoes

Legumes include chickpeas and soybeans. You can add these to a salad or eat legume-rich soups. Legumes and potatoes are good sources of fiber, protein, B vitamins, calcium, iron, and zinc. Try centering a meal on a yam or sweet potato. *Aim for two or more servings per day.* SERVING SIZE: one-half cup of cooked beans; four ounces of tofu or tempeh; eight ounces of soy milk; one large potato.

3. Increase Your Intake of Fruits

Choose whole fruit over fruit juices with little or no fiber. Fruits are full of fiber, vitamin C, and beta-carotene. Don't be afraid of starchy fruits like bananas, which are full of potassium. Aim for a variety of fruits, including those highest in vitamin C, such as citrus fruits, strawberries, and melons. Dried fruit can be enjoyed as an occasional delicacy or a light addition (such as a tablespoon of raisins) to a meal. *Aim for three or more servings per day.* SERVING SIZE: one medium piece of fruit; one-half cup of cooked fruit; four ounces of juice.

4. Increase Your Intake of Whole, Unprocessed Grains

Incorporate brown rice, oat groats, barley, bulgur, millet, amaranth, spelt, and quinoa into your diet. Whole grains are rich in fiber, protein, B vitamins, and zinc. Try building meals around a hearty grain dish. Try sprouted grains for better nutrient usage. Consider sprouted, flourless breads and tortillas. *Aim for five or more servings per day.* SERVING SIZE: one-half cup of cooked grain; one slice of whole-grain bread or one tortilla.

5. Reduce or Eliminate Meat, Poultry, and Seafood

Create meals of legumes, starchy vegetables, potatoes, grains, and leafy green vegetables, with just one to two ounces of lean animal meat or fish if desired. Start with a few plant-based (animal product–free) *meals per week* and gradually work up to many animal product–free *days per week*. You can also try concentrated, vegetarian, high-quality protein sources such as hemp, spirulina, chlorella, and brewer's yeast. These are easy to absorb and can be eaten directly, added to food, or stirred into a drink.

6. Reduce or Eliminate Your Intake of Dairy Products and Eggs

Substitute nondairy alternatives. Try soy, rice, almond, and oat milks. Many frozen desserts too are made from soy, rice, and almonds. Try a tofu scramble for breakfast. Soy cheese is a good alternative for cheese lovers. Just be sure to read the label, since many manufacturers of "plant-based" cheese add casein, a milk protein, to the mix. For serving sizes, follow the labels on these packaged items.

7. Reduce Your Intake of Highly Processed Foods

This group includes such foods as white rice, white flour, and white sugar products: white breads, pastas, cookies, cakes, scones, chips, pretzels, muffins, bagels, crackers, candy, fruit rolls, sodas, milk chocolate, ice cream, and products with high-fructose corn syrup. Less processed, *whole-grain* products, such as whole-grain breads, crackers, and pastas (the label will say *whole* in front of the term *grain*), are a better substitute for the highly processed foods already mentioned. However, if you still tend to feel compelled to eat, or are addicted to, the *less processed whole-grain foods*, stick to the *unprocessed whole grains* themselves, discussed in number 4 of this list. You may have allergic addiction, a topic I discuss in chapter 10. As your chemistry becomes more balanced, you may be able to tolerate some processed whole grains without feeling compelled to overeat them. With respect to sweeteners, choose natural sweeteners like fruits and juices. For natural sugar substitutes, choose stevia, Sucanat, organic blue agave nectar, evaporated cane juice, brown rice syrup, barley malt syrup, blackstrap molasses, and maple syrup, rather than white sugar.

8. Reduce or Eliminate Certain Types of Fats

Avoid artificial fats like margarine, dairy-based fats like butter and cream, and the use of cooking oils and oil-based salad dressings. Fat-free dressings, salsa, and oil-free hummus are good alternatives. Whole plant foods such as avocados, olives, nuts, and seeds have all the fat you need. There are small amounts of fat in grains, vegetables, legumes, and even fruits, so you don't need much more fat in your diet. Try making your own dressing out of avocados, nuts, or whole olives. Nut butters are great on breads, rice cakes, oatmeal, and vegetables. *Aim for no more than two servings per day of healthy fats.* SERVING SIZE: one-quarter cup of raw nuts; two tablespoons of nut butter; four small olives; one-quarter to one-half avocado, depending on size. And don't forget to add two level tablespoons of ground flaxseed each day for your omega-3s.

Eating a handful of nuts or seeds (raw or dry roasted) four to six days a week adds flavor and variety to the diet, and studies have shown that nuts cut health risks. A study of more than eighty-three thousand women found that those who consumed a handful of nuts or one tablespoon of peanut butter at least five times a week were significantly less likely to develop diabetes than those who seldom ate nuts.

About Serving Sizes

Does the concept of serving sizes bring up unhappy memories of dieting and counting calories? If so, don't get too hung up on the serving sizes listed — they're just guides to average servings. Your appetite will be your best guide. So if, for example, you put half a cup of beans on your salad and feel hungry for more, eat more. If you feel hungry for two cups of lentil soup instead of one cup, go for it. If you feel a desire for two nectarines, eat two. Feel free to eat two potatoes instead of one. Just listen to your body's cravings with respect to whole plant foods and eat until you're satiated.

You don't need to weigh and measure your food (or your body, for that matter). Whole plant foods are body balancing. Your body will signal "enough" when you've eaten the right amount. It's unlikely that you'll binge on these foods. I don't think you'll eat ten baked potatoes (without butter and not roasted!) or ten bananas. If these foods are appealing to you, your body is probably giving you a signal that means "more starch, please" or "more potassium, please." Any compulsive cravings — which signal that your body is out of balance — should subside once your body is back in balance.

Generally, it's when we add sugar, refined foods, oil, salt, or dairy products to our diet that we increase the caloric density, trigger the release of powerfully pleasing brain chemicals, unbalance our signals, and end up with strong cravings for more.

The one caveat I add here, as I mentioned in the previous chapter, is that if you have been diagnosed with a metabolic condition such as insulin resistance or diabetes, you may need to reduce your servings of fresh and dried fruits and certain other foods, like white potatoes, that quickly convert to sugar; your body is signaling that there is an imbalance in sugar metabolism. It would be advisable to consult a health care practitioner knowledgeable about plant-based diets to help you with these conditions. An excellent book for addressing these conditions is *Dr. Neal Barnard's Program for Reversing Diabetes*.

Limits versus Deprivation

It's important for all of us to learn to work with limits. In part 1 of this book, I discussed how limit setting is a form of self-love and good self-care. When you allow yourself a small serving of a favorite junk food, you are practicing effective limit setting. Choosing to limit your intake of foods that unbalance your body is a form of nurturance. Telling yourself you cannot ever have a certain food again is a form of deprivation and represents black-and-white thinking. Deprivation feels punitive and is not a loving behavior (unless it's lifesaving, as in, for example, the case of severe food allergies).

There are unhealthy, unwholesome, but tempting, foods around us at all times. Daily we're presented with opportunities to practice limit setting. Rather than fear that one bite or one serving of something will throw off your eating plan entirely and send you on a downward spiral, remind yourself that you can set a nurturing limit in advance and *consciously choose* to have "just one." Then access your willingness to feel all the emotions that surface when you set limits for yourself.

Go at Your Own Pace

Remember, you don't have to make all these changes overnight. Small changes can make you feel more energetic and can reduce your cravings, lower your weight, improve your sleep and mood, and reduce any inflammation you may have. And these positive results will keep you motivated to go further.

There is no rush, unless you create one in your mind. It took you time to get to this place of overweight or poor health, and it will take time to change. You may want to make one change per week, every other week, or one per month. Whatever *feels* right is right for you. You'll need to access your courage to tolerate a bit more discomfort as you make the transition. Remember, you're reading this book because *you're already uncomfortable* with your emotional eating, weight, body image, or health or some combination of these.

Watch the perfectionistic tendency to want to do it all at once. Observe your thoughts. Thoughts such as "I can't make all these changes; what's the use" or "This is just too overwhelming" or "I will be way too uncomfortable" are demotivating and unproductive. Thoughts such as "I can do this, one baby step at a time," "I choose to be patient with myself as I begin to make changes," and "I am willing to be a bit uncomfortable in order to reach my goals" are much more empowering.

Working through any emotional imbalances (by mastering the skills in part 1 of this book) and addressing the brain and body imbalances discussed in the next chapter will make it easier to change your eating habits. If making these changes seems too overwhelming, consider working with a dietitian who specializes in plant-based eating plans, and/or with a professional psychotherapist.

CHAPTER TEN

Principle #3. Address Body and Brain Imbalances

Cara approached me at the beginning of a seminar I was giving on emotional eating. Her words tumbled out in desperation: "I really need your help — I've gained thirty pounds in the last six months and I'm afraid I'll keep gaining. I'm so out of control with food, but I just can't go on another diet. I know my eating is emotional — I feel so overwhelmed. I'm just not sure what to do first."

Cara was a fund-raiser for a large nonprofit corporation, and her days were full of stress. She often skipped daytime meals, ate sweets for an energy boost, and drank coffee and diet soda all day to keep going. Because Cara came home ravenous and drained from work, her night-time meals turned into large, unwind-from-the-day binges. She worked long hours and exercised infrequently because of time constraints and low energy. She struggled with anxiety and depression.

Cara complained of chronic fatigue and irritability and did not feel rested even after a good night's sleep. At times she felt "weak and shaky." Her premenstrual syndrome (PMS) lasted about three weeks of each month — she felt she had only one "good" week per month. Her sugar, carbohydrate, and fat cravings intensified before her period and led to weeks of compulsive junk-food eating every month. She binged regularly on bread, pastries, chocolate, and ice cream.

Her relationship with her parents was also stressful, and Cara felt criticized for her weight and, at thirty-nine years of age, her lack of dating prospects. She felt "too fat" to date, and even though she was terribly lonely, she often turned down social invitations because of her poor body image. She was stuck in a cycle of feeling drained and hopeless, using food for energy, soothing, and comfort — and then feeling more drained and hopeless. It was immediately clear to me that she was struggling with more than just emotional issues.

Cara is representative of the many clients who come to see me for help with their overeating. Like Cara, they are stressed out, depleted, and frustrated. Their bodies are hormonally challenged — adrenal, thyroid, insulin, and sex hormone imbalances are causing sweet and carbohydrate cravings, low energy and fatigue, blood sugar fluctuations, PMS, perimenopausal and menopausal symptoms, overeating, and weight gain. Their brain chemicals are imbalanced, and many, like Cara, have food allergies and are battling food addiction. They feel desperate and don't know where to turn for help.

It's Not Your Fault

Most diet books and weight loss programs fail to address the body and brain chemistry imbalances that fuel overeating. Even the most balanced eating plans can inadvertently trigger body and brain imbalances in sensitive individuals. The majority of clients I work with believe their overeating is emotionally driven. They feel ashamed and guilty about their eating and exercise habits. They see themselves as weak willed and undisciplined when it comes to eating and exercise. And while it's true that most are missing some or all of the self-care skills discussed in part 1 of this book, many are unaware that a significant portion of their overeating may be due to cravings triggered by body and brain chemistry imbalances.

I remind them that it's not their fault that they may have inherited some body and brain imbalances or that they live in a stressful, chemically toxic urban environment. Both can throw off their chemistry. And it's not your fault, either, if you've inherited some imbalances or find yourself living in less-than-optimal conditions.

Change begins with awareness. The first step in resolving the imbalances that lead to overeating is to pay attention to the symptoms. In this chapter, we take a look at the symptoms of hormone and brain chemistry imbalances, food allergies, and food addiction. Once you know what to look for, you can begin to make some simple lifestyle changes to bring your body back into balance. Some symptoms may represent underlying conditions that will require the assistance of a qualified health care provider.

Hormone Hell

Hormones are powerful chemical messengers. They are internally secreted compounds manufactured in specialized endocrine organs. They affect the functions of many other organs and tissues throughout the body. When they are in balance, we feel great. When they are imbalanced, they signal us with various symptoms. We begin our discussion of hormonal imbalances with adrenal exhaustion because as the adrenal glands become overtaxed, other hormonal systems try to compensate. For example, the thyroid can be affected and slow down its output, contributing to fatigue, weight gain, and difficulty releasing unwanted pounds.

Adrenal Burnout

Your adrenal glands sit atop the kidneys, and even though each adrenal is no bigger than a walnut, these powerful glands are responsible for manufacturing life-sustaining hormones like adrenaline and cortisol. These hormones increase your heart rate and blood pressure, focus you, sharpen your senses, release stored energy, and basically prepare you for action. While adrenaline helps you avoid a car crash in a tight situation, cortisol is needed for the longer-lasting stressors, such as illness, trauma, job loss, lawsuit, or divorce. When you're chronically stressed, your adrenals are overworking, producing high levels of cortisol. It's important that cortisol levels return back to normal after stressful events. Constant high levels of cortisol tear down your body in many ways, such as by weakening your immune system and slowing down cellular healing and repair functions. Elevated stress hormones can lead to conditions such as obesity, osteoporosis, and heart disease.

Your adrenal glands also play a role in keeping your blood sugar on an even keel by regulating your reaction to sweets and starches. Too much sugar and adrenaline sounds the alarm: the hormone insulin is sent out to remove the excess sugar from the blood and store it as fat.

Cortisol is also involved in blood-sugar regulation and many other bodily functions, such as the utilization of carbohydrates and fats, the distribution of stored fat, and cardiovascular and gastrointestinal function. Cortisol's anti-inflammatory properties help minimize allergic reactions to substances such as foods, alcohol, and environmental allergens.

When your adrenal glands are taxed, they cannot properly produce other hormones, such as DHEA (dehydroepiandrosterone) — important for many functions, including the growth and repair of protein tissues — and the sex hormones: estrogen, progesterone, and testosterone. During midlife, the adrenal glands become the major source of sex hormone production for both men and women. Adrenal exhaustion is something to take very seriously.

During our first session together, I suspected that Cara was suffering from adrenal exhaustion. She exhibited many of the symptoms of adrenal burnout, which include:

- Cravings for sweets, carbohydrates, and salt
- Weight gain or difficulty releasing weight
- Fatigue
- Feeling tired even with adequate sleep
- Feeling tired after exercise
- Need for caffeine and other stimulants
- Insomnia
- Depression and/or mood swings
- Poor ability to cope — emotionally overwhelmed

- Inability to concentrate; lack of mental alertness
- Hair loss
- Tendency to develop colds and flu
- Headaches
- Low blood pressure
- Dizziness, fainting, or light-headedness
- Heart palpitations
- Symptoms of low blood sugar, such as weakness and shakiness
- Aggravation of allergies
- Sensitivity to cold, loud noise, bright lights, and fumes

Thyroid Imbalance

I also suspected that Cara's thyroid might not be working optimally. Many symptoms of thyroid imbalance are ones already listed for adrenal fatigue. The thyroid gland, situated in the throat area, is a major regulator of metabolism. It produces hormones that regulate food metabolism, energy storage and release, temperature sensitivity, sleep, and more.

There can be many reasons for low thyroid function. First and foremost, you may have inherited a genetic propensity for thyroid dysfunction. Having close relatives with thyroid problems may be an indication of a genetic cause. Both Cara's mother and grandmother had been on thyroid medication for many years, and this was a red flag. Cara also had a history of chronic low-calorie dieting, which can reduce thyroid function. Adrenal fatigue, as well as natural hormonal transitions such as puberty, pregnancy, perimenopause (the ten to fifteen years preceding menopause) and menopause, can affect thyroid function. And some prescription drugs, such as estrogen or lithium, used to treat bipolar disorder, can adversely affect the thyroid. It's important to discuss any drugs you are taking with your physician and your pharmacist so they can determine possible side effects.

Symptoms of hypothyroidism, or low thyroid function, include the following:

- Severe fatigue
- Excessive need for sleep
- Sluggishness in the morning
- Weight gain; difficulty releasing weight
- Depression
- Brittle hair; hair loss
- Brittle nails
- Dry skin
- PMS symptoms; irregular periods; excessive bleeding or cramping
- Lower body temperature; tendency to feel cold
- Low blood pressure
- High cholesterol and triglycerides
- Constipation
- Acne
- Headaches
- Muscle and joint pain
- Reduced sex drive
- Aggravation of allergies
- Poor concentration and/or memory
- Puffy face, feet, or hands; water retention

Unstable Blood Sugar

The cravings for sweets, starches, and stimulants and the fatigue, "weak and shaky" feeling, irritability, and mood swings Cara was experiencing were also possible symptoms of other hormonal imbalances. Insulin is a hormone your pancreas secretes to control blood sugar levels. It moves the sugar out of the blood and into the cells for use in energy production. Too much sugar, refined carbohydrates, and stimulants such as caffeine drive the pancreas to overproduce insulin. This can result in a quick drop in blood sugar called hypoglycemia, leaving you feeling weak, shaky, and drained. Symptoms of low blood sugar include the following:

- Cravings for sweets or alcohol
- Drained, shaky feeling

- Irritability
- Nervousness
- Insomnia
- Dizziness or feeling faint
- Confusion; forgetfulness
- Headaches
- Heart palpitations
- Coordination difficulty
- Blurred vision
- Poor concentration
- Sleepiness
- Depression

Over time, the constant overproduction of insulin can create another condition, called hyperinsulinemia, which can lead to very serious hormonal and metabolic disturbances throughout the body. These include the all-too-familiar insulin resistance that often turns into diabetes. When insulin levels are chronically too high, the body cannot properly break down fat and the result is usually weight gain. Cara's mother had been diagnosed with type 2 diabetes, and I was concerned that Cara might be heading down that road.

Symptoms of high blood sugar include the following:

- Cravings for sweets
- Extreme hunger
- Weight gain
- Increased thirst
- Increased urination
- Vision difficulties, such as blurry vision
- Fatigue
- Irritability
- Unusual weight loss

The Sex Hormones

Our discussion of hormonal balance would not be complete without an exploration of an imbalance in the sex hormones: estrogen, progesterone, and testosterone. Imbalanced sex hormones can cause food cravings, mood swings, low energy, and weight gain at any phase of our lives. Cara complained of her PMS lasting nearly three weeks. It was a no-brainer that her sex hormones were off-kilter.

A large percentage of overeaters I work with have been, like Cara, trying to cope, often unsuccessfully, with the myriad of symptoms they experience as a result of PMS, perimenopause, or menopause. PMS is a complex disorder associated with a wide range of body and brain symptoms recurring fairly regularly during the cycle, followed by a symptom-free phase. Perimenopause is a time when the ratio of estrogen to progesterone in the body can be in a state of flux. A woman is considered to be in menopause when she has not had a menstrual period for one year (which happens, on average, at age fifty-one).

A woman's monthly cycle is under the control of hormones secreted by the ovaries — namely, estrogen and progesterone. Estrogen levels gradually rise the first week or so after her period and peak around mid-month, when ovulation occurs. As estrogen levels taper off and an egg is released, progesterone production begins and dominates the second half of the cycle. Progesterone prepares a woman's body for pregnancy, and if this doesn't occur, the estrogen and progesterone levels fall abruptly, triggering the shedding of the uterine lining and menstruation.

A woman's moods and physical well-being are affected by both of these hormones. When the level of either one is too high or too low or changes abruptly, she may find herself experiencing various unpleasant moods, body symptoms, and food cravings that signal imbalance, especially for sweets, fats, and stimulants.

Symptoms of PMS include the following:

- Cravings for sweet or salty foods
- Increased appetite or thirst
- Weight gain
- Fatigue; cravings for stimulants
- Abdominal bloating
- Breast swelling and tenderness

- Uterine cramping
- Irritability
- Tension
- Headache
- Depression
- Anxiety
- Mood swings or personality change
- Acne or oily skin
- Asthma
- Insomnia
- Constipation or diarrhea
- Change in libido
- Weepiness
- Backache
- Dizziness or fainting

Symptoms of perimenopause and menopause include the following:

- Cravings for sweets, carbohydrates, and caffeine
- Weight gain, especially around the abdomen
- Fatigue
- Water retention; bloating
- Irritability
- Foggy thinking; confusion
- Depression
- Anxiety
- Mood swings
- Hot flashes and/or night sweats
- Inability to handle stress
- Headaches, including migraines
- Menstrual irregularity
- Indigestion, reflux, or flatulence
- Changes in sexual appetite and response
- Low metabolism; thyroid dysfunction
- Unstable blood sugar

- Aggravated allergies
- Sluggishness in the morning
- Insomnia and sleep problems
- Hair thinning and loss
- Infertility
- Vaginal dryness; painful intercourse
- Memory problems
- Low back pain; joint pain
- Diffuse body aches and pains
- Osteoporosis
- Dry eyes; dry skin or wrinkles
- Frequent urination
- Incontinence (urinary leakage)
- Dizziness or vertigo

John R. Lee, MD, Jesse Hanley, MD, and Virginia Hopkins, authors of *What Your Doctor May Not Tell You about Premenopause*, proposed that in America and many other industrially advanced cultures, high-calorie diets full of animal proteins, processed foods, fats, dairy products, sugar, and oils, in addition to environmental toxins, birth control pills, and high stress levels, lead to estrogen levels in women twice as high as those in women of third-world countries, where diets are more heavily plant based. Estrogen levels in men can also be higher.

The authors suggested that when women are fairly inactive and consume many more calories than needed, estrogen production increases dramatically. And our increased exposure to foreign substances called *xenoestrogens*, like plastics, perfumes, and pesticides, that create estrogen-like activity in the body, add to this "estrogen dominance." He believed that American women frequently have estrogen levels that are *too high in relation* to progesterone levels, imbalances directly created by these nutrition and lifestyle factors. The latest research suggests that this estrogen dominance appears to be the cause of many PMS, perimenopausal, and menopausal symptoms and that it is implicated in conditions such as endometriosis, uterine fibroids, and polycystic ovarian syndrome.

Testosterone is the third sex hormone, and it can be unbalanced in both women and men. In women, testosterone imbalance can result in levels that are too high, producing symptoms such as:

- Feelings of aggression or hostility
- Irritability
- Increased sex drive
- Increased facial hair
- Acne

Symptoms of low testosterone in women include:

- Reduced energy
- Mild depression
- Lack of sex drive
- Hair loss
- Dry skin

In men, testosterone can also be imbalanced, with symptoms of low testosterone such as:

- Reduced energy
- Lowered sex drive
- Reduced muscle mass and increased body fat
- Loss of vitality
- Erectile dysfunction
- Thinning hair
- Memory problems
- Mild depression

The main point to keep in mind here is that you need to achieve a harmonious balance of all your hormones. Hormonal balance is complex and ever shifting, and there can be multiple causes of disruption.

Resolving Hormonal Imbalances

If, like Cara, you are experiencing many of the symptoms of the various hormonal imbalances discussed here, it's important to share your findings and concerns with a well-informed health care provider who can test your hormone levels and then diagnose and treat any hormonal imbalance. Always have your hormone levels tested before taking additional hormones or supplements, and retest months later. Saliva testing, which measures active hormones, is considered by many alternative health care practitioners to be the gold standard in testing.

Hormonal imbalance may very well be contributing to your overeating or imbalanced eating. Here are some steps you can take right now to improve your hormonal balance:

- Continue to *add* more unprocessed whole plant foods, especially fresh, raw vegetables, to your diet. Fiber helps move toxins out of the body and fills you up, making it easier to gently release the foods you are consuming that might be contributing to hormonal havoc.
- If you are eating animal products, including eggs and dairy, make sure they are hormone- and pesticide-free, organic, and preferably free-range.
- Continue to significantly reduce or eliminate your intake of processed foods, sugar, and oils.
- Meet most of your daily essential fatty acid requirements with unprocessed, uncooked whole foods such as flaxseed and other seeds, nuts, and soybeans.
- Reduce your use of stimulants like caffeine and nicotine. And reduce or eliminate your use of alcohol, the supercarbo. All of these significantly tax your delicate hormonal balance.
- If you are not exercising, begin to include mild to moderate exercise into your day. If you are overexercising, this can be a stressor. Explore the reasons you are overexercising. In chapter 11, I discuss moving your body.
- Plan more time for adequate sleep and periods of rest in your week — your body needs rest to heal and repair itself. In principle #5, chapter 12, I discuss sleep habits.
- Identify the major stressors in your life, including environmental toxins, and begin to think about ways to reduce them. Later in this chapter, I discuss stress reduction.

Pumping Up Brain Chemicals

Cara's medical tests did confirm that she was in fact suffering from adrenal fatigue and hypothyroidism. In addition, it appeared that she was estrogen dominant, and her progesterone level was very low. Her health care provider wanted to treat her for these conditions first before exploring any underlying brain chemistry imbalance. There was the hope that her moods would clear up as her hormones became balanced. I was concerned that Cara might have an underlying inherited mood disorder, because depression and anxiety ran in her family. She recalled first experiencing depression as a teen, around the time of her first period. Hormonal changes and transitions can often exacerbate underlying mood disorders.

Her use of stimulants and her strong craving for drug-like, highly processed foods artificially concentrated with fat, sugar, and salt (such as chocolate, ice cream, muffins, crackers, cakes, and pastries) were also tip-offs that she might be struggling with both imbalanced brain chemicals and food allergies.

Brain chemistry researchers now understand a great deal about many of the chemicals produced in our brains. They've discovered that brain chemicals called neurotransmitters are released at nerve cell endings, where one nerve cell is near another. These allow messages to pass from one cell to the next and are essential for communication between brain cells. Brain chemicals regulate our mood and mental energy, alertness, focus, and calmness. The quality of our lives is highly determined by our brain chemistry. If it is balanced, our mood generally stays at an even keel and we have good mental energy and focus. Imbalanced brain chemicals can cause many unpleasant feeling states, including anxiety, mania, obsession, phobia, agitation, hostility, depression, weepiness, lethargy, brain fog, confusion, and apathy.

You may be using foods, beverages, alcohol, drugs, and cigarettes to remedy imbalanced brain chemistry: to rev up, focus, lift depression, calm down, reduce anxiety, numb out, and tranquilize. The truth is, you are self-medicating.

Some overeaters tell me that their strongest cravings are for fried foods like French fries and fried chicken and for fatty meats like ribs and bacon. When we discuss releasing these foods from their diet, they tell me they know they should but feel unable to do so. Usually, they believe it's a matter of willpower. Many are relieved when I suggest that they may have some kind of biochemical imbalance in their brains triggering the craving for fatty foods.

Other overeaters purge excess calories after a binge by vomiting or overexercising. Not only does the consumption of drug-like foods provide needed brain chemicals but these two purging activities (symptoms of a condition commonly referred to as *bulimia nervosa*) can also release powerful, soothing chemicals to a biochemically imbalanced brain. These activities can become addictive. Balancing brain chemistry is an important step in resolving your overeating.

Your brain chemicals can become too low or high *occasionally or periodically* from factors such as stress, season changes, drug and alcohol use, poor diet, low-cal dieting, food allergies, and hormonal imbalances. Treatment to restore your chemicals at these times may be all you need. Your brain chemicals also may be too low or high *regularly* from some type of genetically inherited condition. These conditions, usually referred to as *mood disorders*, often require longer-term treatment.

If you try to cope with life's challenges, including your overeating, while your brain chemistry is imbalanced, you will perceive everything as more difficult than it truly is. Once your brain chemicals are balanced, your mood and overall outlook will improve. You will feel more confident, cope with life's difficulties more easily, and have more emotional and physical energy and endurance. And your compulsive food cravings that are the result of brain imbalances will disappear.

The Key Players

An imbalance in any of the following five main mood-related neurotransmitters (brain chemicals) can result in mood disturbances and food cravings:

- Dopamine/norepinephrine
- Glutamine (an amino acid that acts as a neurotransmitter)

- Serotonin
- Endorphins
- GABA (gamma-aminobutyric acid)

Certain brain chemicals keep us feeling energized, upbeat, and alert and help us focus and concentrate. They are like our natural caffeine. Our main energizing brain chemical is called dopamine, and it promotes a sense of satisfaction, drives assertiveness, and pumps up libido. Pleasurable experiences such as lunch with a good friend or a good tennis game tend to elevate dopamine levels. In your body, dopamine converts to another energizing brain chemical, called norepinephrine.

When your brain has enough of these two energizing chemicals, you wake up easily and feel ready to start the day. You have good concentration, attention, and focus, and your energy level is good. And your mood tends to stay at an even keel or be upbeat. Of course, you can be in a bad mood because of factors unrelated to your brain chemistry, but if your brain chemicals are balanced you should feel more capable of handling these stressors.

Caffeine and nicotine increase the release of these energizing brain chemicals and can inhibit their breakdown, keeping you energized longer. If you are highly attracted to these drugs, it may be a sign of low brain-chemical levels. You also may be craving sugar as a pick-me-up because your energizing chemicals are low.

Glutamine is an amino acid, a stimulating, excitatory organic substance that acts as a neurotransmitter. It is critical for optimal brain function, and it boosts our mood, increases alertness, and enhances memory. It also increases libido and facilitates good digestion. Many alcoholics and those who eat sweets compulsively are deficient in this important brain chemical.

Another brain chemical, serotonin, keeps our mood stabilized and contributes to emotional stability and mind focus. This chemical also provides us with a sense of well-being and calmness and helps promote sleep. It is our natural Prozac. Low levels of this brain chemical are associated with depression, excessive weepiness, anxiety, obsessive thinking, phobias, carbohydrate cravings, and PMS.

Probably the best-known of the brain chemicals, morphine-like chemicals called endorphins are associated with "runner's high," relief of pain, euphoria, and the sensation of pleasure (sexual orgasm releases a flood of endorphins). Research has identified more than twenty different types of endorphins. Some compulsive overeaters are also compulsive overexercisers, and this may be due, in part, to low endorphin levels. Those who use food for reward and pleasure may also be low in these chemicals.

GABA, probably the least-known brain chemical, is our natural Valium, and it helps us feel relaxed. If our GABA level is low, we may overeat fatty foods in an attempt to sedate ourselves.

Table 4, "Neurotransmitter Deficiency Symptoms," gives a detailed list of symptoms you may experience if your brain chemicals are imbalanced. You don't have to exhibit all the symptoms listed to warrant an adjustment to your brain chemicals. If you find you have more than a few symptoms in any category, there is a good chance you could benefit from a trial of natural supplements prescribed by an informed health care provider. These include amino acids, essential fatty acids, enzymes, herbs, vitamins, and minerals.

For many overeaters, getting off animal products and heavily processed foods, adding more wholesome plant foods (especially raw vegetables and foods high in amino acids and essential fatty acids), exercising, and reducing stimulant use is enough to correct imbalanced brain chemistry. And if you are having trouble getting yourself to do any of these, imbalanced brain chemistry may be holding you back.

A medical examination must always be the first step in ruling out physical causes of imbalanced brain chemicals, before you begin any supplement or exercise regimen to treat these conditions. Do not stop using any prescription drugs or begin taking any supplements without first consulting your physician.

Table 4

Neurotransmitter Deficiency Symptoms

NEUROTRANSMITTER (BRAIN CHEMICAL)	DEFICIENCY SYMPTOMS	LEADS TO CRAVINGS FOR
Dopamine/ norepinephrine	Increased appetite (especially late afternoon and evening) Fatigue (wake up with low energy or low energy in afternoon) Low mental energy; sluggish thinking Attention difficulties (focus, concentration) Tendency to sleep long hours; may be slow to wake up Low motivation, drive, enthusiasm Apathy, flat mood, boredom, or "the blahs" Tendency to have clutter Tendency to procrastinate Susceptibility to cold; cold hands and feet Tendency to gain weight easily Reduced libido Depression	Sweets Starches Fatty foods Salty and starchy Chocolate Sodas Caffeine Cocaine Amphetamines Tobacco Alcohol Marijuana Aspartame
Glutamine	Fatigue Low mental alertness Unclear thinking Low mood Imbalanced blood sugar Poor digestion	Sweets Starches Alcohol
Serotonin	Tendency to compulsively binge; food obsession Anxiety, worry, panic attacks Irritability, agitation, crankiness Impulsiveness Little or no sense of well-being Negativity	Sweets Starches Chocolate Wine Marijuana Tobacco

(continued)

Table 4
Neurotransmitter Deficiency Symptoms (continued)

NEUROTRANSMITTER (BRAIN CHEMICAL)	DEFICIENCY SYMPTOMS	LEADS TO CRAVINGS FOR
Serotonin (*continued*)	Obsessive thoughts and compulsive behaviors Phobias Perfectionism; need for control Sensitivity to light or seasonal changes Attention difficulties Poor sleep Fibromyalgia Lack of libido Depression	
Endorphin (20+ different types)	Tearful; overly reactive to emotional or physical pain Anxiety Phobias Tendency to engage in addictive, pleasurable activities (e.g., running, gambling, sex)	Sweets Starches Chocolate Opiates Alcohol Marijuana Tobacco
GABA	Anxiety Difficulty relaxing Stiff or tense muscles Exhaustion from stress Excessive reactions to normal stressors	Sweets Starches Alcohol Marijuana Valium

Food Allergy and Its Sidekick, Addiction

We all have our favorite foods. For me, freshly baked bread tops the list. And for some of us, once we start eating these foods, we can't stop — it's as if they're calling to us. Before we know it, we've eaten the *whole* loaf of bread or polished off the entire carton of ice cream or bag of cookies. Even though we may overeat other foods too, these particular foods we feel compelled to eat and may even be addicted to them.

If you tend to eat certain foods compulsively, there's a good chance that you're allergic to them. When you think of allergies, you probably think of unpleasant symptoms such as hives or rashes. But did you know that not all allergic reactions are unpleasant? You may in fact feel better after eating allergenic foods. This reaction is called allergic addiction. In an attempt to soothe the irritation caused by allergic foods, your body releases powerful soothing brain chemicals. Over time you can become firmly addicted to these pleasurable chemicals. Allergic symptoms and food addiction are important signs of imbalance.

Many popular diets include food allergens in their eating plans. Given this and the fact that their caloric allotments are too low, it's no wonder people can't stick with them. To be successful, any program addressing overeating must address food allergy and food addiction.

So what exactly is a food allergy? It's an adverse reaction to a particular food. Generally a person's response is considered an allergy rather than a sensitivity if the food in question causes an immediate, measurable immune-system reaction. Food sensitivities (also known as delayed food allergies) involve the immune system too, and tend to cause reactions anywhere from forty-five minutes to several days after ingestion. The difference between the two is really just a matter of degree. There is considerable debate in scientific and medical circles about how to define these terms, because often a person's symptoms are not accompanied by *any* measurable level of antibodies. If your body keeps giving you signals in the form of symptoms, though, you most likely have some sort of sensitivity even if your allergy tests show that your responses are in the normal range.

Your immune system's job is to recognize and destroy anything perceived to be foreign and harmful: viruses, bacteria, molds, poisons, and even cancer cells. It's a sophisticated system made up of many different types of cells designed to combat a variety of invaders.

Whenever your body encounters an allergen, your immune system becomes activated and releases a flood of substances called allergy mediators. One of these substances, histamine, is familiar to most of us. Its job is to expand blood vessels, which causes inflammation, overproduction of mucus, and, with them, discomfort. (This is why we take antihistamines.) We may experience this inflammation as a runny nose, sneezing, itchy eyes, nausea, vomiting, diarrhea, or even clogged airways.

While most of the time the immune system doesn't get stimulated to action by the foods we eat, in allergy-prone people the immune system mistakenly goes after normally harmless substances, like peanuts or strawberries. (See the sidebar "Common Causes of Food Allergy.")

Clear, strong, and immediate reactions to foods, such as rashes, hives, and wheezing, make for an open-and-shut case, and you will gladly choose to avoid the foods that cause these symptoms. But other unpleasant symptoms that you may be familiar with can also be signs of food allergy. These include compulsive food cravings, water retention, irritability, foggy-headedness, fatigue, sinus problems, headaches, bloating, stomachaches, constipation, depression, hyperactivity, anxiety, and arthritis. Table 5, "Symptoms of Food Allergy," gives a comprehensive list of these signs.

Common Causes of Food Allergy

MOST COMMONLY CAUSE ALLERGIES	OFTEN CAUSE ALLERGIES	
Wheat	Alcohol	Peanut butter
Milk	Cane sugar	Coffee
Soy	Buckwheat	Coconut
Corn	Berries	Mustard
Eggs	Oranges/citrus fruits	Yeast
Fish	Chocolate	Coloring agents
Shellfish	Tomatoes	Preservatives
Peanuts	Nightshades	Nitrates
Tree nuts	Peas	Pesticides
	Pork	

Source: Adapted from Sharon Faelten, *The Allergy Self-Help Book* (Emmaus, PA: Rodale Books, 1983), p. 25.

Table 5

Symptoms of Food Allergy

AREA AFFECTED	POSSIBLE SYMPTOMS	AREA AFFECTED	POSSIBLE SYMPTOMS
Body Weight	Water retention Weight gain (or loss)	Digestive Tract	Bloating Constipation Diarrhea
Ear, Nose, and Throat	Copious mucus Coughing or wheezing Earache Ear infections Ear itching/ringing Hoarseness Sinus inflammation Sneezing Sore throat Stuffy nose		Flatulence Heartburn/reflux Irritable bowel Nausea Rectal itching Stomachaches Ulcers
		Muscles and Joints	Arthritis Pain Poor coordination Stiffness Weakness
Eyes	Blurry vision Dark circles Itchiness Puffiness Wateriness	Bladder and Genitals	Bed-wetting Bladder discomfort Frequent urination Genital discharge Genital itch Infertility Urgent urination
Head	Dizziness Headaches, including migraines Slurred speech Vertigo	Energy	Fatigue Food cravings Hyperactivity Lethargy Restlessness Sleepiness Sluggishness
Skin	Acne Dryness Hives Profuse sweating Rashes		
Mouth	Canker sores Dry throat Inflammation of lips, gums, tongue, or mouth		

(continued)

Table 5			
Symptoms of Food Allergy (continued)			
AREA AFFECTED	POSSIBLE SYMPTOMS	AREA AFFECTED	POSSIBLE SYMPTOMS

Chest	Achiness or pain
	Asthma
	Bronchitis
	Congestion
	Difficulty breathing
	Heart palpitations/
	  irregular heartbeat
		Attention and Memory	Attention difficulties
			Confusion/foggy
			  head
			Learning challenges
			Poor concentration
			Poor memory

Sleep	Difficulty falling asleep
	Insomnia
	Poor quality of sleep
	Waking up too early
		Mood	Aggressiveness/
			  hostility
			Agitation/
			  irritability
			Anxiety
			Compulsions
			Depression
			Mania
			Mood swings
			Obsessions
			Phobias

The allergist Theron Randolph, MD, was one of the original proponents of the theory of allergic addiction. He warned that continued consumption of food allergens eventually make you ill. The ingestion of food allergens not only chronically overtaxes a person's immune system but can also lead to nutritional deficiencies as a result of chronic inflammation of the gastrointestinal tract and malabsorption of nutrients.

William H. Philpott, MD, and Dwight K. Kalita, PhD, authors of *Brain Allergies*, suggest that foods of all kinds, as well as chemicals such as food additives, pesticides, and herbicides, can qualify as "addictants." The allergy-addiction cycle goes something like this: Once we ingest the food, it stimulates our immune system, which produces allergy mediators, like histamine, as well as powerful, soothing, opiate-like brain chemicals.

We notice an immediate good feeling, even while our body may be experiencing some mild discomfort, such as a headache or stomachache (and some symptoms of allergy may be delayed). Within minutes or hours, we notice a strong craving for the substance again. We may experience other withdrawal symptoms, such as irritability or agitation, depression, lack of concentration, or anxiety. We ingest the food again and obtain relief. This state of temporary relief is called addiction.

When we continue to ingest food allergens on a regular basis, we generally experience some chronic allergic symptoms. This eventually overtaxes our immune system and disrupts our metabolism, which can result in weight gain, inflammation throughout the body, and chronic disease. While many of these symptoms could be caused by conditions other than allergies, it would be wise to explore the possibility of a food allergy with your health care provider or by home testing, if you experience any of these symptoms on a regular basis.

Identifying Food Allergies

From both personal and professional experience, I've noticed that three of the most common food allergens seem to cause the majority of allergy symptoms: wheat, sugar, and dairy products. Many packaged foods include all three, and many weight loss programs provide prepackaged meals including these items. Allergies to these three foods can cause compulsive cravings and overeating, sabotaging the best of intentions.

WHEAT

The seeds or grains of grasses like wheat, oats, rye, barley, spelt, and triticale all contain a family of proteins called gluten. These proteins can be difficult to digest and may inflame the digestive tract of sensitive individuals. Wheat tends to be the most troubling grain, especially when it's highly refined into flour. Many clients I work with crave and consume flour products multiple times per day. They also report symptoms such as bloating, water retention, low energy, fatigue, sleepiness, sinus problems, body aches, PMS, anxiety, depression, and poor concentration. Many gluten-sensitive individuals can tolerate sprouted grains or whole grains, such as oats or barley, without symptoms but notice an aggravation of symptoms if the grains are processed at all. Highly sensitive individuals may do better with low-allergy, unprocessed grains like brown rice or quinoa. You may also want to avoid grains completely for a period of time and instead consume low-allergy starchy vegetables like yams, sweet potatoes, and winter squash.

SUGAR

The standard American diet includes sugars extracted from many basic food sources, such as sugarcane, corn, barley, and beets. Refined sugar has no nutritional value; it's unnatural for us to eat or drink these extracted sugars. Complex carbohydrates and fruits provide your body with all the natural sugar it needs.

Food manufacturers add sugar to just about everything — breakfast cereals, crackers, breads, frozen goods, catsup, soup, pickles, sauces, and so on. Read the labels and you'll be surprised. Too much sugar produces an inflammatory response and wreaks havoc on your digestive system and metabolism. Sugar is also highly acidic and throws off your acid-alkaline balance. It's not a girl's best friend, either, because it ages the body. The constant energy lift, insulin surge, and intoxication you get after ingesting sugar can lead to addiction and create imbalances in your body and brain chemistry.

In susceptible individuals, too much sugar can lead to yeast cell overgrowth, a condition called candida albicans. Yeast infections are unpleasant and often hard to get rid of. And an overgrowth of yeast cells means more sugar cravings, as these hungry little beasts like sugar.

DAIRY

The milk of any animal contains opiate-like chemicals that provide an infant with a feel-good sensation encouraging it to drink more. Food manufacturers sell milk and condensed-milk products such as cheese, ice cream, and yogurt, which produce this same sensation in the consumer. These foods can cause an allergy-addiction cycle in sensitive individuals. They also may cause common allergy or sensitivity symptoms such as digestive upsets, respiratory difficulties, and inflammation in general. And despite what you've heard, milk is not the best source of calcium. Pasteurization of dairy products destroys enzymes in them that are essential for our absorption of calcium. Plant foods such as beans and green leafy vegetables, like kale, collard, mustard greens, and broccoli, are much better sources.

While wheat, sugar, and dairy products tend to be the most common food allergens, there are many other foods, such as eggs, corn, fish, and soy, that can cause allergy and need to be investigated.

Treating Food Allergies

Food allergies can be a lot more challenging to identify than allergies to airborne substances, drugs, or even cosmetics. Many physicians admit that conventional skin tests and blood tests (radioallergosorbent testing, or RAST) are unreliable or less reliable for food than, say, for dust or pollen. Symptoms do not always fall into predictable, easily observed patterns. And there is often a delay in the onset of symptoms, ranging from minutes to days, making it difficult to trace the cause. Symptoms may come on slowly after many years of daily ingestion of particular foods to which you are sensitive.

There are other tests your health care provider can run that can be a bit more effective in identifying allergies. These are the enzyme-linked immunosorbent assay, or ELISA, test or a family of blood tests known as the antigen leukocyte cellular antibody test, or ALCAT, which measure allergic response to various panels of allergens, including foods, chemicals, molds, and other substances. Saliva testing can identify allergies to all gluten-containing grains and cow's milk protein.

Many alternative health care practitioners utilize a technique called Nambudripad's Allergy Elimination Technique (NAET) to aid in the identification of allergens. Utilizing applied kinesiology, a trained practitioner performs muscle testing to determine whether allergic substances are weakening the body. (Visit www.naet.com to find a practitioner in your area.)

In my practice I encourage clients to test themselves at home first by monitoring symptoms and eliminating or rotating suspected foods, as this is a highly effective way of identifying food allergies. By eliminating foods, rotating foods, or eating troublesome foods only at widely spaced intervals, you can keep most food allergens from reaching the critical point and triggering symptoms. Make a special note on your Daily Eating Log of any of the symptoms you experience that are listed in table 5, especially food cravings, fluid retention, and inflammation, three common indicators of food allergies. With respect to inflammation, look for symptoms such as joint aches and pains, arthritis, clogged airways, runny nose, sore throat, swollen lips, itchy or puffy eyes, headaches, and foggy-headedness.

If you have many bothersome allergy symptoms, and your Daily Eating Log contains allergy foods, especially the top three, it would be best for you to follow an elimination diet, which is a way of home testing for food allergy. On the elimination diet, you avoid the primary suspect, such as wheat, in all its forms, for one to four weeks (go as long as you can) to see how you feel. If the idea of eliminating any food makes you very upset or unhappy, this is probably a good indication of food allergy and addiction.

An allergist I worked with more than twenty-five years ago used to have a simple, effective rule for identifying possible food allergies. He said that if you *love* a particular food and feel *very* resistant to removing it from your diet, there is a good chance you have an allergic addiction to it. The love affair is actually a flood of pleasing brain chemicals released from the intake of allergens. I loved anything with flour, dairy, or sugar — bread, pasta, pizza, muffins, pretzels, scones, cookies, candy, chocolate, cottage cheese, ice cream, cheese, yogurt, and so on. I enjoyed fruit, brown rice, potatoes, corn, and starchy vegetables; I did not *love* these foods.

Once you've eliminated a particular food for one to four weeks, you eat the food again, in generous portions at several meals in one day, and note your symptoms. If your symptoms return, it's generally a good indication that an allergen is present. It's best to take one food at a time when you are testing a food and following an elimination diet. The first few days off these favorite foods may be difficult as you experience withdrawal symptoms. But within four to five days you should feel better.

If you feel so attached to particular foods that you absolutely cannot eliminate them, the next best step is to try a rotation diet. The most common rotation diet is the Four-Day Rotary Diversified Diet, developed by Dr. Herbert J. Rinkel in 1934. On this plan you eat the offending food only once every four days, trying to eat as little of it as possible on that day. This allows the level of antibodies in your system to subside a bit before encountering the offending food again. It will help to reduce your cravings and some of the unpleasant physical symptoms you're experiencing, while still allowing you to look forward to your favorite foods. This may also allow you to determine the minimum amount of an allergen that you can safely consume without triggering symptoms. Any sense of deprivation you may feel can be reduced by continuing to add to your diet wholesome, unprocessed plant foods that you enjoy.

If you feel extremely resistant to eliminating or rotating certain foods, this may be an indication that your hormones and/or brain chemicals are imbalanced. When these imbalances are corrected, you will find it easier to gently release these foods from your diet.

A couple of months into working with her health care provider, Cara noticed she was feeling much better. "I'm finally getting a good night's sleep, and I wake up feeling rested. Since I'm not so tired during the day, I'm less irritable, and everyone's noticing that. I'm also a lot more efficient at work, so I can leave at a decent hour. I hired a personal trainer, and I'm actually enjoying exercise. And I feel energized after working out. Oh, and my PMS is so much milder and lasts less than a week now."

While Cara was no longer bingeing, she still noticed that she felt addicted to caffeinated beverages and foods containing flour, sugar, and dairy. Once again, my hunch was that Cara was having a difficult time releasing these substances because of low brain chemical levels and the presence of food allergies.

Her health care provider agreed, and Cara began a supplement regimen that included amino acids, herbs, essential fatty acids, vitamins, and minerals. Within a few weeks, Cara noticed that she could more easily turn away from the foods to which she normally felt addicted. She was able to follow an elimination diet for one month, getting rid of flour, sugar, and dairy products. And it was easy for her to stop drinking caffeinated beverages because once her brain chemicals were better balanced, she felt too hyped up when she drank regular coffee or tea.

Even though Cara's body and brain were becoming much more balanced and she had lost some weight, she still noticed the desire to occasionally use food for comfort and soothing. But now that she had more psychological and physical energy, she was motivated to practice the self-care skills presented in part 1 and tackle her emotional and physical stressors.

Chronic Stress Can Lead to Emotional Eating

We are all aware that we need to reduce stress. We cope daily with demanding jobs, traffic, noise, financial and social pressures, caregiving duties, and relationship challenges. Lack of sleep and exercise, unhealthy convenience foods and beverages, chronic dieting, and illness or infection put our bodies to the test. Traumatic events and significant losses max out our emotional and spiritual reserves.

Chronic stress taxes our endocrine system, imbalances our body and brain chemistry, and overloads our coping mechanisms, leading to an emotional appetite and an exaggerated craving for comfort and energy.

Stress in small doses can be useful; it can motivate us to make necessary changes and to be productive. The stress you feel before running a 5K race can be energizing and motivating. Sometimes financial pressure or job dissatisfaction is the necessary stressor that gets you to change jobs or go back to school. Too much stress, though, and we become imbalanced. Our bodies are not designed for constant stress.

Even though we can never eliminate stress altogether, the goal is to stay in balance. We want to manage our lives in such a way that we enjoy our work and relationships, create time for relaxation, and have the endurance and resilience to meet life's challenges, without turning to food for support.

Stress management begins with identifying your stressors. For simplicity's sake, I like to divide stressors into internal and external stressors. In part 1, we explored the internal (emotional) stressors, such as chronic depressive, anxious, and lonely feelings; negative, self-defeating thoughts; and ineffective coping patterns like perfectionism and acting out. In chapters 8 and 9 we looked at how chronic dieting and modern drug-like foods can be additional sources of internal stress. In this chapter, we've further seen how imbalanced body and brain chemistry causes internal stress. In the next two chapters we'll take a look at additional internal stressors: sedentary lifestyles and poor sleep.

In this section, let's explore external stressors that directly lead to poor food choices and emotional eating. Even if you're choosing healthy foods, you may still be eating to cope with stress. External stressors can be broken down into two categories: personal and nonpersonal stressors.

External Stressors

PERSONAL	NONPERSONAL
Overwhelming responsibilities	Economic downturns
✦ caregiving duties	
✦ provider duties	Noise
✦ community service	
	Traffic
Health challenges	
✦ self or loved ones	Trauma, e.g., robbery, rape, shootings, accidents, earthquakes, tsunamis
Financial challenges	
	Societal compliance responsibilities, e.g., tax filings, jury duty, lawsuits
Relationship challenges	
Losses	Environmental toxins
	✦ pollution and fumes
Trauma, e.g., abusive parent, spouse	✦ pesticides/herbicides
	✦ additives/preservatives
Job pressure	✦ molds
✦ long hours	✦ cleaning solvents and products
✦ late-night shifts	✦ chemical exposure, e.g., paint, asbestos, hair dye, nail polish
✦ difficult relationships	
✦ difficult assignments	✦ cosmetics and perfumes

Take a moment and make a list of your external stressors. Divide your list of stressors into those you feel you have no control over and those you may be able to alter, avoid, or change. Sometimes just the act of writing down all your stressors can motivate you to take stress seriously and begin to reduce it.

Strategies for Handling Stressors

External stressors often feel outside our control. Some, such as an economic downturn, a job layoff, or the serious illness of a loved one, cannot be prevented or avoided. When you can't prevent, alter, or avoid a stressor, you must find a way to accept it, adapt to it, and cope with it *for now*.

STRESSORS OUTSIDE YOUR CONTROL

- Allow yourself to feel and express all your emotions regarding the stressor. Writing them down in your journal can help you express pent-up emotions and reduce the tendency to reach for food.
- Share your emotions with an empathic family member, friend, counselor, or therapist. Even when there is nothing you can do to change a stressful situation, sharing with others can be a big stress release.
- Watch any tendency toward catastrophic thinking. Reframe any self-defeating thoughts and repeat the uplifting, hopeful thoughts over and over. (Review skill #2, in chapter 3.)
- Practice mind-quieting relaxation techniques such as breath counting and yoga. (I discuss these techniques in part 3.)
- Try to take a longer-term perspective. Will this stressor be gone or reduced in a month, six months, or a year? Remind yourself regularly that this will not last forever. If it is a longer-term stressor, like the terminal illness of a loved one, remind yourself that your feelings and acceptance level are going to change with time. Good mental health requires courage, frustration tolerance,

resilience, endurance, and the ability to delay gratification — all skills you can and must learn and practice.

- Look for the positives. Has this stressful situation provided any opportunities for learning and growth? Has it made you stronger and more resilient? Has it helped you become more empathic? If you're feeling bitter, resentful, and victimized, and you can't see any positive outcomes, see this as a sign that you are still processing the stressor, or that it may be triggering old pain that needs to be worked through. (Review skill #3, in chapter 4.) You will move toward acceptance at your own pace.

- Shift your focus. Take some time to reflect on all the wonderful things in your life. This includes your health, traits, talents, and accomplishments; the loved ones in your life, including furry friends; and even basic things like a roof over your head, clothing, a hot shower, and food.

- Adjust your expectations. Life can throw us a lot of curve balls. Just when things are going great, you're in a major car accident. Just when you launch your children and have time for yourself, you shift into a difficult and challenging menopause. This is not what you expected! Life constantly requires us to be adaptive, adjust our expectations, create a new "now," *and* get on with our lives. Not always easy to do.

- Add more joy. While you are going through this stressful time, see if you can add more time for relaxing and enjoying. Take a bath, get a massage, garden, read a good book, and don't forget to laugh.

STRESSORS WITHIN YOUR CONTROL

- Assess your limits. If you feel overwhelmed by responsibilities, evaluate honestly and realistically what you can and cannot handle while still maintaining balance. Consider relinquishing some responsibilities, putting them off, or even changing some habits, such as ordering groceries online.

- Practice saying no to added responsibilities. This may require you to feel new, uncomfortable feelings such as guilt and anxiety about not being a good friend, daughter or son, wife or husband, community participant, and so on. Or the feeling you're missing out on some activity.
- Assess your personal boundaries. Do you feel too enmeshed or merged with the needs and feelings of others, or do you feel too cut off and isolated from other people? Loose or rigid boundaries can be a source of stress. (Review skill #4, in chapter 5.)
- Reevaluate relationships that cause a lot of stress. Do you have a toxic or difficult close relationship in your life? Can you limit your exposure to this person? Do you need to end a relationship that is no longer beneficial?
- Seek professional help for dealing with trauma, losses, disappointments, and difficult relationships. There is no reason to try to do it all by yourself.
- Consider a course in assertiveness training to help you take charge of challenges and address problems head on.
- Consider a course in time management to help you learn to prioritize responsibilities and tasks, realistically schedule time, reduce to baby steps anything that is overwhelming you, delegate responsibility, and create a more balanced schedule.

Reducing Environmental Stressors

Many of us are living in toxic urban environments today. While we may not be able to eliminate all environmental stressors, there are actually many things we *can* do to reduce their impact. Consider the following:

- If traffic stresses you out, try changing your driving times or routes, if possible. Join a carpool or explore mass transit.
- Exercise outdoors during low-pollution hours.
- Buy organically grown fruits and vegetables to avoid pesticides and herbicides.
- Read food labels and avoid foods with unnatural additives.

- Get rid of mold if you're aware it's a problem.
- Replace traditional household cleaning chemicals with green versions.
- Limit use of plastic wrap and containers that leach hormone-disrupting chemicals.
- Wear a mask when you paint.
- Avoid air fresheners, flame retardants, and bug and plant sprays, and find green alternatives.
- Review cosmetics, hair-care products, and sunscreens for hazardous ingredients such as hormone-disrupting petroleum-based chemicals.

Keep in mind that reducing and managing stress is a process. Trying to reduce all your stress at once only adds more stress. Start with changes that are easy to make, like switching to green cleaning products or changing your driving route. Applaud yourself for the willingness and courage you have to examine your life and make changes.

CHAPTER ELEVEN

Principle #4. Move Your Body

What comes to mind when you think about exercise — something enjoyable that you *want to* do to satisfy a natural need to go out and move your body? Or does exercise feel like something unpleasant you *have to* do to burn calories, maintain your weight, firm up, and stay healthy? For sure, exercise may be the last thing you feel like doing when your body isn't functioning well because you're stressed out, sleep deprived, or overweight. And if you're dieting and cutting too many calories or skimping on carbohydrates, it's unlikely you'll have the energy needed to exercise.

When you're not exercising regularly, you may feel disconnected from your body signals and ignore early warning signs of illness. Without sufficient exercise, your muscles and bones will weaken and deteriorate and you can easily pull muscles doing simple routine activities. And you'll be more susceptible to colds and flu, because your immune system is not as strong. Our signals work best when our machine is operating optimally, and this requires movement.

Sure, physical activity increases your metabolic rate, helps you burn calories, and relieves stress. But did you know that it also helps regulate your appetite, enhances your metabolism of fats, and appropriately lowers hormone levels like insulin and excess estrogen? And the benefits of exercise extend far beyond weight management. Regular physical activity can increase your energy, regulate your mood, help reduce the risk for several health conditions and diseases, and improve your overall quality of life.

Whether you're a want-to or have-to exerciser, if you're having trouble starting or sticking with an exercise plan, the first step will be to correct any body and brain chemistry imbalances addressed in the previous chapter. If you're sleep deprived, you'll want to read about that in chapter 12.

And if you still can't get yourself to exercise, I'll help you take a look at your excuses and overcome your resistance to moving your body.

It's always a good idea to talk to your doctor before beginning any new physical activity program, especially if you have any chronic conditions such as diabetes, high blood pressure, a heart condition, or arthritis.

How Much Exercise Do We Need?

Many of us today get much less physical activity than our parents or grandparents did. They raked leaves, shoveled snow, chopped wood, scrubbed floors, hand-washed garments and hung them to dry, hand-mowed lawns, washed and waxed cars, and often walked miles per day. And for our earliest ancestors, physical activity was a natural way of life. They didn't think about exercising and fitness. Roaming and working the land, gathering food and water, cutting firewood, and securing shelter supplied plenty of physical exertion.

Granted, it would be difficult to make physical activity a natural way of life today. Our jobs often require long commutes by car and sitting at desks most of the day. But we can *easily* add more regular physical activity to our daily lives. The good news is that our bodies are adaptive, and even if we haven't been exercising for quite some time, our body systems will improve quickly once we get moving. We don't have to use high-tech equipment or join noisy, crowded gyms. And exercising doesn't need to be hard, boring, supersweaty, or challenging.

The American College of Sports Medicine updated its physical activity guidelines for healthy adults in July 2011. The college recommends that adults include four different types of activity in their exercise routine: cardiorespiratory, resistance, flexibility, and neuromotor exercises.

Cardiorespiratory Exercise

Cardio exercise, important for a healthy heart and weight management, consists of any type of exercise that increases the work of the heart and lungs. The best cardio exercises for you are the ones you'll actually do, day in and day out. It's most important to choose activities you enjoy and mix up the activities to prevent boredom. The college's recommendations for cardio exercise are as follows:

- Adults should get at least 150 minutes of moderate-intensity exercise per week.
- Exercise recommendations can be met through 30–60 minutes of moderate-intensity exercise [like brisk walking] five days per week, or 20–60 minutes of vigorous-intensity exercise [like jogging, running, or cycling] three days per week.
- One continuous session and multiple shorter sessions (of at least 10 minutes) are both acceptable to accumulate desired amount of daily exercise.

Remember, as the third bullet point above suggests, you can reach your goal of thirty minutes of moderate-intensity physical activity per day by breaking it up. It's just as effective to exercise two times per day for fifteen minutes each time or three times per day for ten minutes. This could mean a brisk ten-minute walk before breakfast, at lunch, and before dinner. Or ten minutes on the treadmill in the morning and twenty minutes before dinner. *Anyone* can create this kind of time in his or her schedule.

Many activities, such as swimming or bicycling, can be either moderate or vigorous in intensity, depending on the level of effort applied. With moderate-intensity exercises, you should notice an increase in your heart rate but should still be able to talk comfortably.

Examples of moderate-intensity activity include the following:

- Walking at a brisk pace (3 mph or faster)
- Slow jogging or hiking
- Ballroom and line dancing
- Water aerobics
- Bicycling slower than 10 mph
- Light downhill skiing
- Skating and blading
- Pilates or Gyrotonic classes
- Baseball or softball
- Tennis (doubles)
- Working out with exercise videos
- Scrubbing floors
- Mowing the lawn
- Shoveling snow

Examples of vigorous-intensity activity include the following:

- Race walking
- Running
- Stair climbing
- Cross-country skiing, vigorous downhill skiing
- Hiking uphill or with a heavy backpack
- Swimming laps
- Bicycling more than 10 mph or up steep hills
- Tennis, mainly singles
- Competitive sports: basketball, soccer, football, hockey
- Martial arts
- Fast rope-jumping
- Aerobic or fast dancing
- Rowing
- Continuous lifting and moving of furniture
- Heavy gardening (digging or hoeing)

Resistance Exercise

Since muscle tissue is metabolically more active than fat, you can keep your metabolism revved up by including strength-training exercises in your routine two or three days per week. Train each major muscle group using a variety of exercises and equipment. The goal would be to complete eight to ten strength-building exercises, with eight to twenty repetitions per exercise. You can accomplish this at home or at the gym with a small array of weights or exercise resistance bands, a bench, an exercise ball, or even just your own body weight — for example, by doing sit-ups, squats, push-ups, and pull-ups. You could do these exercises during television commercials or even when talking on the phone. You just need to get creative.

If you're just beginning this type of exercise, you'll probably need some instruction. A series of private sessions with a personal trainer or an ongoing class with an instructor should give you the basics.

Flexibility Exercise

Stretching increases the flexibility of joints and muscles and helps prevent injuries. Tight, inflexible muscles or constant injuries are a sign that you're not stretching enough. Don't forget to include some stretching exercises two or three days per week to improve your range of motion. Each stretch should be held for ten to thirty seconds. Repeat each stretch two to four times for each major muscle group. Again, television time is a good time for stretching — I do my stretching exercises during the nightly news.

Neuromotor Exercise

And as if these guidelines weren't enough, the American College of Sports Medicine added to the mix a fourth category of exercises, sometimes called functional fitness training. Exercise in this category involves motor skills such as balance, agility, coordination, and gait and includes activities designed to improve physical function and muscle awareness and to prevent falls in older adults. The college recommends working out for twenty to thirty minutes per day, two or three days per week, doing multifaceted activities like yoga, tai chi, Pilates, Gyrotonic, and balance-ball work.

Don't Forget to Warm Up and Cool Down

Take three to five minutes at the beginning of any physical activity to go slow and properly warm up your muscles before you increase the intensity. Also, a few minutes before stopping the activity, cool down by decreasing the intensity and lowering your heart rate.

Before You Get Overwhelmed . . .

I know the guidelines I've outlined here can feel daunting. But in actuality, it's not that hard to meet them, even with the busiest of schedules. It just requires a little planning. Let's look at a few examples of client workouts to get an idea of how to cover all the bases.

Keep in mind that your body was meant for movement — moving a half hour or more per day is natural; sitting morning, noon, and night is not.

Jenny's Weekly Workout Schedule	
MONDAY AND WEDNESDAY	15-minute walk before and after work (equals 30 minutes); 20-minute resistance routine after evening walk; 10 minutes stretching during nightly news
TUESDAY	Yoga class at the gym before work
THURSDAY	Pilates class after work
FRIDAY	30-minute walk before work, plus stretching
SATURDAY	Rest day with some light housecleaning
SUNDAY	1-hour bike ride or walk, plus stretching

Tonya's Weekly Workout Schedule	
MONDAY AND THURSDAY	20-minute run before work; 20-minute resistance routine, plus 10 minutes of stretching
TUESDAY	20 minutes of balance-ball exercises before work
WEDNESDAY	Gyrotonic class after work
FRIDAY	Rest day
SATURDAY	30- to 60-minute hike, walk, or bike ride
SUNDAY	Gentle stretching plus light gardening
Leslie's Weekly Workout Schedule	
MONDAY AND THURSDAY	Boot camp before work (includes walk/run 30 minutes plus 30 minutes of resistance and stretching exercises)
TUESDAY	15-minute walk before and after work (equals 30 minutes)
WEDNESDAY	20 minutes of yoga stretches in the evening
FRIDAY	15-minute stationary bike ride before and after work (equals 30 minutes)
SATURDAY	30-minute DVD exercise video (includes resistance, balance, and stretching)
SUNDAY	30-minute water aerobics or dance class

Excuses, Excuses — So What's Stopping You?

Okay, now you know what you *should* do in terms of exercising. So what's keeping you from exercising? As a certified personal trainer with twenty-five years of experience designing exercise programs, I've heard all the excuses, I always take them seriously, and I can get anyone moving.

"I'm Too Tired to Exercise"

If you feel too tired to even start exercising, or you find that you feel more tired and drained *after* exercising, it may be a sign that your diet is not supporting you and/or your thyroid or adrenals are taxed. You'll need to boost and support these hormonal systems first, as discussed in the previous chapter. Even though you may not be ready to embark on an exercise regimen, you can start increasing your activity a bit by doing the following:

- Park farther away from work or stores.
- Take the stairs instead of the elevator; even one flight will help.
- Increase the amount of your activity around the house: vacuuming, raking leaves, scrubbing floors, mowing the lawn, washing the car.
- Stand up and lift small hand weights during television commercials or while on long telephone calls.
- Dance to your favorite music.
- Work in your garden.
- Clean out the garage.
- Walk your dog.
- Perform gentle stretching, yoga, or calisthenics exercises.

"I Don't Have Time to Exercise"

If you feel you don't have time to exercise, you'll need to evaluate your priorities. Just like brushing and flossing, exercise is a way of taking care of yourself. And since you can break it up into two or three ten-to-fifteen-minute sessions each day, there's no reason you can't find time.

If your life is very busy with work and taking care of children or parents, you'll have to be creative. My client Jane, a wife and the mother of two young children, found that stopping on her way home from work to walk around the park for half an hour provided some nice time to wind down before the evening's caretaking duties. Sandra, a busy executive, found that she could easily carve out ten minutes for a brisk walk at lunch on the days she didn't have appointments, as well as take a twenty-minute walk in the early morning or after work.

"I Hate to Exercise — It's Boring and Uncomfortable"

When clients tell me exercise is boring, I suggest they find activities they enjoy. You don't have to join a gym, run, swim, or ride a bike to get fit.

Take a Zumba dance class, play sports on a team, go hiking with a group, take tennis lessons, or try water aerobics. Try exercising with a friend; or if you can afford to, hire a personal trainer.

If, in general, you just don't enjoy moving your body, focus on selecting activities that are tolerable, and then periodically vary them so you'll keep exercising over the long haul. You'll need to build up your tolerance for discomfort. Try to replace negative thoughts about exercising with positive reframes, such as "I feel good when I take better care of myself" or "Exercise helps me reduce stress" or "I can get myself to do *anything* for ten minutes."

"It Doesn't Make a Difference in My Weight"

Do you find yourself thinking, "It doesn't make a difference in my weight unless I do intense cardio for a half hour or more and sweat a lot — and I'm too out of shape to do that"? Do you have a tendency to stop and start exercise programs? Perhaps you associate exercise with dieting and weight loss — you begin exercising at the start of a diet and stop exercising at some point when you stop losing weight, get bored, or life gets busy. If you're like my client Louise, you try to do too much exercise too soon and quickly burn out.

When I asked Louise, who hadn't exercised for quite some time, to commit to exercising in the upcoming week, she agreed and offered up a frequency and intensity *way* too high for her first week. She committed to taking a brisk half-hour walk each day for at least five days. I suggested that starting with this much might cause her to be too tired or feel like a failure if she couldn't accomplish it. "How about starting with walking two or three times this week for ten to fifteen minutes per session?" I asked. Her response was typical of the perfectionism that emotional eaters tend to display: "That's not enough — it will hardly make a dent in my weight. And that's pathetic; I used to do so much more."

Don't get stuck in the trap of thinking that it doesn't count unless it's vigorous, goes on for a long time, and causes you to sweat. Research has shown that moderate-intensity activity that raises your heart rate, and that is broken up into increments as short as ten minutes each, is enough.

By taking it slow, Louise would have less soreness and less risk of injury, and this would reduce the chance of her feeling like a failure or feeling unmotivated. By forgoing the gratification of watching the pounds come off fast, she would increase her capacity to tolerate frustration. She would learn to set realistic goals and effective limits for herself. These self-care skills, covered in part 1 of this book, set the stage for sustained weight loss.

Let me suggest that you separate exercise from weight loss. I know that exercise helps you lose weight, but you need to keep exercising long after you've lost those unwanted pounds. So it's best to separate the two and slowly begin an exercise regimen that you can comfortably stick with. This will involve changing the type of exercise periodically to keep it fun and interesting, and increasing the intensity if it gets too easy. And don't forget to keep adding a bit more activity into your daily life, like taking the stairs and parking farther away from work or stores.

"It Reminds Me of Being Pushed to Exercise by My Parents and Teachers"

Perhaps you don't want to exercise because of old, unpleasant associations, such as being forced to run around the track in grade school, feeling uncoordinated in gym class, or being ridiculed by your father on the tennis court. If you find you're extremely resistant to exercising, make a list of the reasons you don't want to exercise or any negative associations you have from the past regarding exercise. Share these with a friend or therapist. Often this is enough to get you started.

It's important to find activities *you* enjoy and to do it just for yourself. Try to focus on how you feel *after* you move your body: your energy level is better, you feel less stress and have more self-esteem, you sleep better, and you have less fear of disease.

Set Realistic Goals

Once you've explored all your excuses, it's time to set some realistic exercise goals. Keep in mind that you don't have to immediately achieve all the recommendations made by the American College of Sports Medicine. Set a plan for the upcoming week that you are sure you can achieve. Remember that it's better to *do less to start* and to feel positive about your accomplishment. Use your Daily Food Log or a separate journal or calendar to record your daily or weekly activities. It can be highly motivating to log your progress. Write down each day's activities, along with one statement regarding the benefit you're receiving from exercise. For example, "Walked 15 minutes. Exercise is helping me lower my blood pressure and feel better about my body."

Eating for Exercise

You'll need lots of wholesome carbohydrates to fuel your exercise sessions. Choose unprocessed carbohydrates like fruits and grains before working out. The general rule is carbohydrates before exercise; after exercise, eat foods that take longer to digest (proteins and fats).

Listen to your body's signals to know what and how much to eat before a workout and how soon after eating you can comfortably work out. Everyone's body is different. Experimenting with different foods before and after exercise will help you identify what works best for your body.

Overdoing It

Overexercising is a stressor and can result in adrenal exhaustion and hormonal imbalance. It also throws off your acid-alkaline balance, leaving you at risk for degenerative conditions such as osteoporosis. Quality rest is just as important as exercise.

How do you know if you're overexercising? The general signs to watch out for include the following:

- Feeling exhausted soon after exercise or the next day
- Waking up feeling unrested after plenty of sleep
- Having difficulty sleeping
- Dreading exercise
- Having soreness that doesn't quickly go away
- Experiencing a more frequent need for stimulants such as caffeine or sugar to get going

A small percentage of exercisers become addicted to exercise and ignore their bodies' signals for rest. In addition to having imbalanced brain chemistry, most people who compulsively overexercise have emotional imbalances that have led to their obsession with exercise. Having trouble managing depression and anxiety, structuring time, or coping with a sense of inner emptiness; experiencing difficulty in setting reasonable limits; and dealing with perfectionism, a fear of fat, or a distorted body image — these are all examples of emotional imbalances that can lead to overexercising. Mastering the self-care skills discussed in part 1 of this book is a good start in addressing these emotional imbalances.

CHAPTER TWELVE

Principle #5. Sleep to Satiation

It's 11 PM New York time, and Emily is sitting in front of her brightly lit computer screen while finishing up some work, answering emails, and enjoying a dish of ice cream. As she heads to bed at 11:45, she turns on the television to begin winding down. Propped up in bed with a book in hand, the light blaring, and the television glaring, she falls asleep. At 6 AM she awakens to the loud buzz of the alarm clock. She hops out of bed, groggy, plugs in the coffeemaker, and gets on the treadmill for a half hour of exercise before the hectic morning begins. What's wrong with this picture?

It's 8 PM California time, and Emily's sister, Deb, is just putting the kids to bed. At 8:30 she turns on the television and gets on the stationary bicycle for her half hour of exercise. Her husband, John, is working late at the office, and it's the only time she could fit in exercise today. At 9:15 she showers, then heads to the kitchen to wash the dishes and make lunches for the next day. John arrives home around 9:30, and Deb prepares a sandwich for him. Hungry from exercising, she eats half a sandwich herself. At 10:30, munching on stale jelly beans, she turns on her computer to check the kids' activity schedule for the next day and researches designs for her daughter's upcoming birthday party invitations. At 11:15 she finds John in bed watching a movie. She turns on her bright bedside light and proceeds to finish the chapter in the book she started last night. At 3 AM John gets out of bed and turns off the lights and television. They had both fallen asleep with the lights on and television blaring. At 5:45 Deb is awakened by her youngest daughter, who isn't feeling well and is running a fever. What's wrong with this picture?

Both Emily and Deb would like to lose weight. Both struggle with daytime fatigue, low energy, and overeating. Both are chronically sleep deprived and are routinely overriding their bodies' natural cues for rest and sleep. They are exposing themselves to bright lights, noise, activity, and food at times of the day when their bodies require dim light, quiet, rest, and sleep. Overeating and weight gain are common side effects of the lack of sleep.

Sleep and Weight Gain

Have you ever noticed how much hungrier you are when you don't get enough sleep? Sleep is often the first thing we give up when we're short on time. In a world of increasing stress, deadlines, and 24/7 connectivity via cell phones and the Internet, it seems that there just aren't enough hours in the day. And yet adequate sleep is one of the most important aspects of weight maintenance and good health. When we're sleep deprived, we often turn to food rather than sleep to boost our low energy levels.

Mounting evidence suggests that lack of sleep has multiple effects that can all result in weight gain. Sleep is a biologically active time. Repair, maintenance, and detoxification functions all occur when you sleep. When your internal clock is disrupted, it may throw off many bodily functions, including metabolism, hormonal balance, brain chemistry, cognitive function, and immunity. Chronic sleep deprivation may lead to irritability, anxiety, and depression — all contributors to emotional eating.

A 2006 study at Case Western Reserve University in Cleveland examined the sleep habits of over sixty-eight thousand women. Researchers found that the women who had slept less than five hours a night were

32 percent more likely to gain thirty-three pounds or more over the course of the sixteen-year study than the women who had slept at least seven hours a night.

The more you sleep, the better your body can regulate the chemicals that control hunger and fullness. Scientists have found that long-term sleep loss interferes with the body's endocrine system by triggering increased insulin resistance and a disruption of appetite-regulating hormones. Lack of sleep leads to a rise in ghrelin, the hormone that turns on hunger, and to a restriction in leptin, the hormone that makes you feel full. When we are sleep deprived, we eat more because we are actually hungrier. We are also awake more hours, and since we are often sedentary during that extra waking time, we consume more calories than we burn. Voilá, weight gain.

The Sleep Robbers

It's somewhat of a no-brainer to say that substances containing caffeine, like coffee, tea, chocolate, cola drinks, and certain over-the-counter medications, will keep you up at night. Some people can drink a cup of coffee and go right to sleep, but most of us will experience disrupted sleep from the use of stimulants. Caffeine can stay in your system for as long as fourteen hours. It increases the number of times you awaken at night, decreases your total sleep time, and affects the quality of your sleep.

Nicotine, like caffeine, can also stimulate the release of excitatory brain chemicals and inhibit the natural production of sleep-inducing hormones. While it acts as a sedative at low doses, at high doses nicotine causes arousal during sleep.

You may also want to think twice about that glass or two of wine in the evening. While alcohol may initially help you relax, it can cause nightly arousal as it is metabolized and cleared from your system. Headaches, sweating, and intense dreaming are all common with alcohol use. While you may not be aware of how alcohol disrupts your sleep, ask yourself if you feel refreshed, or groggy and hung over, when you awaken.

Have you noticed that certain foods affect your ability to get a restful night's sleep? While light carbohydrate snacks may be sleep-inducing because of the effect they have on serotonin levels, it's best to stay away from heavier meals near bedtime — they can lead to digestive disturbances and poor sleep. And while your sleep and overall health may be enhanced by supplementing your diet with multivitamins, minerals, or amino acids, be careful not to take stimulating vitamins (the Bs) and amino acids too late in the day, since they may affect your sleep.

When the Sandman Is Nowhere in Sight

Any of us can have a sleepless night or two, but when it happens regularly for more than a few weeks, it's considered chronic insomnia. When there are no contributing physical or psychological conditions, it is usually brought on by poor sleep hygiene — habits conducive to getting the right amount and quality of sleep. In addition to the poor sleep habits previously discussed, low-level anxiety and stress can easily rob us of a good night's sleep. Many of my clients complain of not being able to "turn off their minds" at night. I generally suggest that they use a journal earlier in the evening to put troubling feelings or thoughts on paper and take them off their minds before bed. Remind yourself that you can think of them tomorrow and that you have control over your mind. It's also a good idea to avoid having stimulating conversations an hour or so before bed. Natural sleep aids such as valerian root and herbal teas can be calming.

Chronic insomnia can also be the result of a medical or psychological illness. Physical conditions contributing to sleeplessness include hot flashes and hormonal fluctuations associated with perimenopause and menopause, diabetes, sleep apnea, restless leg syndrome, urinary incontinence, fibromyalgia, arthritis, chronic pain, bipolar disorder, and generalized anxiety disorder. Chronic insomnia is a health alert — your body is trying to tell you something, and you need to pay attention and take it seriously. It's best to address this type of insomnia with your health care provider.

Let There Be Dim Light

It appears that before Thomas Edison's discovery of the lightbulb, our ancestors slept about nine to ten hours each night. Without artificial light, they went to bed not long after dusk and awoke at dawn.

Deep within the brain is our internal clock, a powerful cluster of nerve cells that produce hormones that regulate our sleep-wake cycle. Exposure to artificial or natural light stimulates the release of excitatory stimulating hormones like cortisol. With fading light, our bodies begin to produce the sleep-promoting hormone melatonin.

Artificial light, while a wonderful invention, throws off our natural circadian rhythm. When we turn on artificial light at night to stay up and read, watch television, work on the computer, eat, or exercise, our body produces stimulating hormones, making it more difficult for us to unwind and easily fall asleep. This can overtax our adrenal glands (the makers of cortisol), further contributing to our daytime fatigue, overeating, and weight gain.

If you are having difficulty getting quality sleep, consider adjusting your habits. Try exercising earlier in the day or refrain from partaking in stimulating activity in bright light in the evening. Prepare for bed by calming down and dimming the lights one to two hours before bed. If your bedroom has too much light, consider blackout shades and even an alarm clock without a light. Maintaining a quiet, dark, and comfortable sleep environment will offer the best chance for restful sleep.

Get Your Full Dose of ZZZs

While individual needs may vary and there are no hard-and-fast rules, the National Sleep Foundation, a U.S. educational and scientific nonprofit organization dedicated to improving sleep health and safety, recommends that most adults get seven to nine hours of sleep per night. Anything below or above that amount may carry health consequences for some individuals. The amount of sleep you need may be less or more — it's the amount *you* need to feel rested, refreshed, and alert.

Just as our bodies use finely calibrated hunger and fullness mechanisms to regulate our caloric intake, they also have sleep mechanisms that regulate our rest and sleep. If we are exercising vigorously, our bodies will encourage us to get more sleep by adjusting our desire for it. Similarly, our bodies will signal an accumulating sleep debt with symptoms such as grogginess, daytime fatigue, decreased work performance, irritability, and health complications like weight gain. If you can, it's best to pay back any short-term sleep debt quickly by sleeping in to catch up, going to bed earlier, or napping. Long-term cumulative sleep deprivation may have serious health consequences, including heart disease and obesity.

Just as we are designed to eat to satiation, we are also meant to sleep to satiation. The best way to determine the average amount of sleep you need is to allow yourself to sleep to satiation as often as possible. This means sleeping until you spontaneously wake up, without the aid of an alarm clock. You'll need to set a bedtime early enough to allow you to sleep as long as you need. Once any sleep debt is paid off, you'll settle into your natural sleep pattern.

Filling Up Spiritual Reserves

PART THREE

Filling Up
Spiritual
Reserves

CHAPTER THIRTEEN

When Overeating Is Driven by Spiritual Hunger

If you're reading this part of the book, most likely you sense that some deeper longing or hunger within you is fueling your overeating. The concept of spiritual hunger resonates with you. You're longing for more of something in life, even if you seem to have everything you once desired. While you long to put an end to your overeating and have a slimmer, healthier body, a part of you knows that even *that* won't make you truly happy. Something is missing, and you can't quite put your finger on it.

Once you've begun to master the self-care skills covered in part 1 and to follow the body-balancing principles offered in part 2, it's easy to fall prey to the illusion that weight loss and better health will solve all your problems. After all, when your self-esteem has improved, and you feel better emotionally and physically, and your clothes fit better, haven't you arrived at your goal? Yes and no.

Often when we reach our goals, we find that their achievement brings little *permanent* satisfaction. We may begin to wonder if there is more to life than pursuing our endless earthly desires. Symptoms such as emptiness and restlessness may represent a spiritual hunger that can ignite our emotional eating.

The skills and practices you've put in place so far have paved the way for the third and final component of your journey toward mind, body, and spirit wholeness: spiritual connection and fulfillment.

In our everyday lives we're usually concerned with acquiring something, striving for some condition, or connecting to some being. As overeaters, we're particularly concerned with our appearance, weight, health, pleasure, and comfort. It's easy to get caught up in the materialistic life and lose sight of our spiritual needs.

Just as a wholesome meal nourishes the body, spirituality nourishes the soul. We all desire a life filled with purpose and passion, a life rich in soul-nourishing connections to family, friends, community, animals, and nature. The spiritual component of well-being involves a search for meaning, serenity, and joy that goes beyond our day-to-day concerns.

An enduring sense of peace, happiness, safety, and security cannot be found in things, conditions, or beings. It can't be found in perfect beauty, health, wealth, or loving attachments. At any point, we can experience setbacks and losses. The peace, happiness, safety, and security you seek are already within you; you need only make contact with your inner reserves.

Thomas Moore, an inspiring theologian, a psychotherapist, and the author of the *New York Times* bestseller *Care of the Soul*, suggests that "a spiritual life of some kind is absolutely necessary for psychological 'health.'" I couldn't agree more. He writes, "In the broadest sense, spirituality is an aspect of any attempt to approach or attend to the invisible factors in life and to transcend the personal, concrete, finite particulars of this world. This spiritual point of view is necessary for the soul, providing the breadth of vision, the inspiration and the sense of meaning it needs."

Spirituality means something different to each individual. For some, it involves regular religious practice. For others, it may involve a personal, individualized practice that fosters connection to a benevolent guide or force. And still others experience spirituality as a deeply felt heart connection, sense of awe, and gratitude. For many, the concept itself is a turnoff because they equate spirituality with organized religion and this conjures up unwanted and long-discarded dogmas and rituals from childhood. Some equate the topic with unfounded and ungrounded New

Age, otherworldly practices. If you are one of the many who bristle at the mere mention of spirituality, or you find that the topic overwhelms and confuses you, let me suggest that you think of spirituality in terms of care of your soul, as defined by Thomas Moore: " 'Soul' is not a thing, but a quality or dimension of experiencing life and ourselves. It has to do with depth, value, relatedness, heart and personal substance." He also states, "A soulful personality is complicated, multifaceted and shaped by both pain and pleasure, success and failure. Life lived soulfully is not without its moments of darkness and periods of foolishness."

Are Your Spiritual Reserves Depleted?

How do you know if your overeating represents a spiritual hunger or "call from your soul" telling you that something is out of balance? You can start by asking yourself if you experience any of the following symptoms of spiritual depletion on a regular basis:

- Emptiness
- Restlessness
- Unease
- Purposelessness
- Meaninglessness
- Lack of inspiration or motivation
- Boredom
- Loneliness or a sense of aloneness
- Longing for there to be more to life
- Lack of personal fulfillment
- General sense of discontentment or dissatisfaction
- A sense of being lost in life

Setting Aside Time to Care for Your Soul

The five practices introduced here are for everyone, regardless of religious affiliation or spiritual orientation. They will assist you in filling up your spiritual reserves and taking the best care of your soul. Setting aside time to consciously shift your focus away from daily concerns will allow you to gain a more expansive perspective on your life and access a sense of peace and joy you may have never known before. This joy has absolutely nothing to do with your beauty, weight, possessions, or attachments or whom you know. This joy can put an end to your emotional eating.

The Five Soul-Care Practices

In part 1 of this book, I stated that the primary cause of your emotional eating is your disconnection from yourself. And I meant what I said. But once you have reconnected to your authentic *feeling self* and have built a kind and loving internal world, your work may not feel complete. There may still be a sense of disconnection causing your eating. You may feel disconnected from the deeper reserves of joy, passion, and contentment within or from your higher self or higher power. You may feel disconnected from other nourishing human beings or from nature. Or perhaps you feel disconnected from your calling or sense of purpose in life.

Even when we've achieved our desired weight loss and improved our health and our lives seem relatively full, we can still experience symptoms of spiritual depletion. The five soul-care practices that follow will assist you in addressing this disconnection and filling up your spiritual reserves:

Practice #1. Quiet your mind.
Practice #2. Practice letting go.
Practice #3. Fill your life with purpose and meaning.
Practice #4. Fill up on nourishing connections.
Practice #5. Practice gratitude.

In this section of the book, you'll discover:

- how to stop focusing on daily concerns and quiet your mind with simple, time-tested practices;

- how to stay in the present and stop living in the past or the future;
- how to access a storehouse of inner treasure more nourishing than any meal;
- how to let go of your illusions of control that lie behind your beliefs about happiness and contentment;
- how to release attachments that no longer serve you;
- how to create a more purpose-filled, meaningful life;
- how loneliness is bad for your health;
- how social connection regulates your physiology;
- how to attract nourishing others into your life;
- how to enhance your spiritual connection; and
- how the mindfulness practice of gratitude can open your heart and fill up your reserves.

While this book was designed for you to proceed from part 1 to part 3, if you're beginning with this part of the book, keep in mind that mastery of the self-care skills in part 1 will make it easier to put the five soul-care practices into place. It may be more difficult to address higher-level needs when your most basic needs have gone unmet for a long time and are clamoring for attention.

CHAPTER FOURTEEN

Practice #1. Quiet Your Mind

Do you ever feel like a human *doing* rather than a human *being*? Our daily lives can be so hectic and stressful. Many of us start our days in a rush, jolted awake by a noisy alarm clock and a strong cup of joe. We wolf down a breakfast or grab food on the run and make our way through noisy, heavy traffic with angry, frustrated fellow commuters. We arrive at our workplace and rush through the day feeling overwhelmed by the sheer volume of work to do, problems to solve, and deadlines to meet. Perhaps we skip breaks and eat a quick lunch at our desk just to get through the workload.

Then it's back into the traffic so we can run errands, hit the over-crowded gym, get home, prepare dinner, meet family and social obliga-tions, and go to bed in time to get enough rest to do it all again tomorrow. And then there's the weekend, where we pack in as many errands and as much pleasure, including food, as we can before the workweek begins. Whew! Sound familiar?

Our stressful lifestyles can leave us feeling chronically anxious and overwhelmed. Our thoughts race and our mental chatter never lets up. We overeat, drink, or distract ourselves in an attempt to feel calm. Even though you may not be able to reduce the multitude of tasks you have to accomplish in a day or all the roles you play, you *can* minimize their negative effect on your mind, body, and spirit. You can do this by consciously withdrawing from your busy schedule to quiet your mind and replenish your soul's reserves.

All spiritual traditions encourage some form of silent retreat from the workaday world. The goal of any retreat is to move away from our current concerns and fears, relax, and connect with a quiet, serene, peaceful place within ourselves. We all have this calm place inside. It is the center of our being. There is a storehouse of inner treasure there for us to claim.

As we make repeated contact with this long-lost part of ourselves, our vitality and zest for life increase. And our ability to relate and love is enhanced. When you sit down to quiet your mind, it may feel like you're taming a wild horse. Your mind is not used to being reined in, and it will go to great lengths to avoid your control. With practice you can gain mastery over your thoughts and train your mind to be still. You can choose to retreat; turn off the television, computer, and phone; and carve out time to center and calm yourself. It's up to you; it's your choice. You don't have to be a victim of your noisy mind or pressurized environment.

You may be thinking, "I can't do this." The place of calm inside you seems inaccessible. Perhaps you've tried to quiet your mind, but it seems like a lot of work and near impossible. I have no doubt you can quiet your mind. You just need to access your willingness to *consistently* engage in experiential practices that allow you to become still. And you need not spend a lot of time doing it, burn incense, chant "Om," or sit in the lotus position (unless, of course, you want to). Ten minutes or more per day in a comfortable position and a quiet place are all you need.

Time-Tested Practices

Many different techniques are available for quieting the mind. Just as there is no universal exercise program, there is no one *right* program or technique that works for everyone. Any practice you choose must fit your unique emotional, intellectual, and sensory style. The goal with each technique is to completely involve and focus your whole being on an activity.

You gently and continuously bring your attention back to the activity. The following four techniques are particularly helpful for beginners:

Technique 1. Breath-counting meditation
Technique 2. One-pointed attention
Technique 3. Mantra repetition or chanting
Technique 4. Yoga

Technique 1. Breath-Counting Meditation

In this variation of a Zen Buddhist exercise, you try to focus your complete attention on counting your breaths. Thoughts, emotions, and sensations come and go; you notice them without judgment and return your focus to your breathing and counting.

It's best to close your eyes when you are beginning this exercise so there is less distraction. Set a timer for five minutes. Set a goal of doing this meditation exercise daily, if possible. Of course, you can increase the time if that feels appropriate.

STEP 1. FIND A QUIET, PRIVATE, COMFORTABLE PLACE

Sit upright on a comfortable cushion, chair or couch; lying down leads easily to falling asleep. Wear loose, comfortable clothing. Make sure you turn off anything that might distract or interrupt you.

STEP 2. FOCUS ON YOUR BREATHING AND COUNTING

As you inhale deeply, count the number *one* to yourself silently and then exhale deeply. Repeat this three times, counting up to the number *four*, focusing solely on inhaling, exhaling, and counting. When you exhale on breath four, begin counting with the number *one* again. You can breathe through your nose or mouth, whichever is most comfortable.

STEP 3. BREATHE IN QUIETUDE, BREATHE OUT TENSION

As you inhale, imagine yourself breathing in light, love, peace, and calm. Breathe out and exhale stress, negativity, and worry. Focus on how it feels as the air moves through your nostrils, mouth, and chest. Your body and mind are beginning to relax. You are calm, quiet, safe, and still in this moment.

Technique 2. One-Pointed Attention

This is a good technique to use when you find yourself worrying or obsessing about something and unable to stop thinking about it. Most of us have little mastery over our thoughts, especially fearful, anxious, or worrisome ones. Daily thoughts about fears, self-doubts, losses, mistakes, disappointments, and comparisons can haunt us and rob us of joy. Every time we recycle these thoughts, we become more anxious and depressed. We attempt to distract and comfort ourselves with food, shopping, television, and the like, but the bothersome thoughts pop right back up. They quickly deplete our spiritual reserves of vitality, peace, and calm.

You cannot live in quietude if your thoughts are unmanageable and unruly. Used in a variety of mystical schools, one-pointed attention is a technique you can use to train your mind to be focused and still. Eknath Easwaran, author of *Meditation: Commonsense Directions for an Uncommon Life*, writes, "In meditation we train the mind to be one-pointed by concentrating on a single subject — an inspirational passage. Whenever the mind wanders and becomes two-pointed, we give more attention to the passage, and we do this over and over again. It is certainly challenging work, but gradually the mind becomes disciplined, taking its proper place — not as the master of the house, but as a trusted, loyal servant whose capacities we respect."

This technique has been called the "meditation of contemplation" because it involves concentrating on a single subject actively and dynamically, without talking. There are many ways to practice this technique. You can even focus your attention on a single object, such as a seashell or leaf, rather than an inspirational passage. I recommend beginning this exercise with a passage or prayer that inspires you, because it not only helps you still and focus your mind but also has the added benefit of imprinting on your consciousness words that can transform your fear and insecurity.

One of my favorite inspirational passages is the Prayer of Saint Francis of Assisi. You need not practice any particular religious faith to find this inspirational passage appealing. You can replace the words *Divine Master* or *Lord* with *my highest self* or *my wisest self* if that works better for you.

Lord, make me an instrument of thy peace.
Where there is hatred, let me sow love;
Where there is injury, pardon;
Where there is doubt, faith;
Where there is despair, hope;
Where there is darkness, light;
Where there is sadness, joy.

O Divine Master, grant that I may not so much seek
To be consoled as to console,
To be understood as to understand,
To be loved as to love;
For it is in giving that we receive;
It is in pardoning that we are pardoned;
It is in dying [to the self] that we are born to eternal life.

Set a goal of practicing this technique daily, if possible, or at least a few times per week. Plan to practice one-pointed attention fifteen minutes or more per session.

STEP 1. FIND A QUIET, PRIVATE, COMFORTABLE PLACE

Sit upright on a comfortable cushion, chair, or couch. Wear loose, comfortable clothing. Make sure you turn off anything that might distract or interrupt you.

STEP 2. SLOWLY READ THE WORDS OF THE PASSAGE

Concentrate on one word at a time, hearing the sound of each word in your mind as you concentrate on the meaning of the passage.

STEP 3. TRY NOT TO LET YOUR MIND WANDER

At times, this will be difficult. Your mind will create associations with the words, and you will notice you are far away, deep in thought. Gently refocus your attention on the passage. Notice how relaxed and peaceful you feel when you focus your mind.

Technique 3. Mantra Repetition or Chanting

To many, the ancient word *mantram*, or its popular variant *mantra*, conjures up the idea of mystical, foreign, Far Eastern practices. The word *meditation* does too. Easwaran explains,

> A mantram is a spiritual formula of enormous power that has been transmitted from age to age in a religious tradition. The users, wishing to draw upon this power that calms and heals, silently repeat the words as often as possible during the day, each repetition adding to their physical and spiritual well-being. In a sense, that is all there is to a mantram. In another sense, there is so much! Those who have tried it — saints, sages, and ordinary people too — know from their own experience its marvelous potency.

Some common generic mantras include the following:

Aum or Om (said to be the vibrational sound of the universe)
Peace
Love
All is One

Here are some classic spiritual or religious mantras:

Hail Mary (Catholic)
Baruch Atah Adonai or the Shema (Jewish)

Hare Krishna or Hare Rama (Hindu)
Om Namah Shivaya (Hindu)
Om Mani Padme Hum (Buddhist)
Allahu Akbar (Islamic)

The mantra technique consists of chanting, or rhythmically repeating, a word or phrase over and over again. As with the previous two techniques, the goal is to focus attention, do only one thing at a time, and still the mind. Over a long period, regularly repeating the mantra enables you to gain mastery over your turbulent, ever changing mind.

Initially, it's best to sit quietly and practice mantra repetition for five to fifteen minutes. Over time, you can repeat the mantra anywhere, anytime. You can use the mantra to calm your agitation when you're anxious, angry, or fearful. Try repeating the mantra to quiet your restless, wandering, impatient mind when you are waiting for a red light to turn green or are in line at the grocery store. Try lulling yourself to sleep by repeating the mantra before bed. This is a surefire way to fall asleep with a still, peaceful mind.

STEP 1. FIND A QUIET, PRIVATE, COMFORTABLE PLACE

As in the previous two techniques, make sure you sit upright on a comfortable cushion, chair, or couch. Wear loose, comfortable clothing. And remember to turn off anything that might distract or interrupt you.

STEP 2. BEGIN REPEATING THE WORD OR PHRASE ALOUD

Find a comfortable rhythm and stick with it. You can repeat it slowly or quickly, as you like. You may want to download or purchase a CD with a chant that inspires you.

STEP 3. WHEN YOUR MIND BECOMES DISTRACTED, GENTLY BRING IT BACK TO THE MANTRA

After a few weeks of daily mantra practice, you may want to increase the time to twenty or thirty minutes. As you keep working on disciplining your mind so that it focuses solely on the mantra, you will notice there are increasingly longer periods of time when you are aware of nothing but the mantra. At last, your mind is in the present moment, free and at peace.

Technique 4. Yoga

Yoga is a centuries-old philosophy and practice brought to us from the East. Here in America, we tend to be drawn to yoga as a physical practice for balancing and healing the body. But one of yoga's main benefits is that it brings quiet, clarity, and focus to the mind as well. The word *yoga* has many translations, including "union," "joining," and "uniting," which describe the integration of body and mind that represents yoga's essence.

In the West, yoga is typically associated with hatha yoga, a form of physical discipline that utilizes many asanas, or postures, and breath work. Within the system of hatha yoga are numerous schools, such as Iyengar, Ashtanga, Bikram, and even power yoga.

You do not have to believe in any spiritual or mystical philosophy to benefit from yoga. All you need to do is practice the poses and pay close attention to your breath and body as you continuously adjust your alignment and balance. Although your mind will wander, yoga forces you to bring your mind back to the pose and focus on your torso, limbs, muscles, and joints.

The best way to learn yoga is with a teacher. A good teacher can see imbalances that you are unaware of (because they feel normal to you) and help you push past emotional blocks and physical resistances. Often, the poses you resist or avoid are the ones you most need to do.

Begin by trying a few different types of classes to find the practice and teacher that best suits your needs and temperament. If you take an Iyengar yoga class, you'll generally hold poses longer and pay closer attention to alignment than in some other schools of yoga. Props like blocks and chairs may be used to accommodate special needs. If you try a Bikram yoga class, your muscles will be thoroughly warm as you perform a series of poses in a near-hundred-degree, sauna-like room. This yoga experience involves sweating and moving toxins out of the body.

It's best to practice yoga regularly. Once you are familiar with the poses, aim to practice for ten to fifteen minutes at least every other day. And remember to practice patience with yourself as you embark on this path to body, mind, and spirit wholeness.

Keep Your Expectations Realistic

Be prepared to have good and bad sessions with the mind-quieting practices I've discussed here. One day you'll feel like you're in the flow and everything is going well. The next day, your mind will be racing, your body restless, and it will feel like you're just going through the motions. This is all part of the process. The key is to stick with the practice. It may be helpful to keep a journal of your daily or weekly mind-quieting practices and experiences so you can see your progress. Over time, your mind and body will become well-trained servants, and peace and harmony will be your reward.

CHAPTER FIFTEEN

Practice #2. Practice Letting Go

M ost of us believe that if we apply enough effort and do the "right" things, we can control our lives. If we have the talent, ability, or good fortune to manifest many of our desires, we become, without realizing it, invested in this *illusion*. We dream big, set goals, and become emotionally attached to power, beauty, money, prestige, material possessions, people, and even the idea that things will *always* go our way.

Jenny, a forty-two-year-old mother and a caring physician with a busy family medicine practice, subscribes to the superwoman philosophy. She believes a woman can have it all — a satisfying career, home life, children, community involvement, good self-care — *and* do it all well. She is a devoted health care provider, an adjunct university professor, and a member of many professional boards. She is a loving, involved mother, good friend, and wife and helps care for her aging parents.

Jenny is frustrated with her inability to lose weight, as well as her inability to get pregnant again. She hopes to have a second child before it's too late. "Having it all" is part of Jenny's *illusion of control*; she believes she *should* be able to attend to all her responsibilities, eat healthfully, exercise, and get enough sleep. Yet she grabs unhealthy food on the run, drinks caffeinated ice tea all day to keep going, exercises infrequently, and rarely sleeps more than six hours per night. She has little to no quality downtime. In frustration she told me, "I hate to admit this, but I'm often impatient with my staff, daughter, husband, parents, and even my patients."

Jenny is skilled at manifesting her desires, and she feels a general sense of control in her life. But her inability to lose weight is a constant source of frustration and shame and an overt sign, she believes, to herself and the world that she is out of control. Her inability to maintain a healthy body weight and a patient, pleasant attitude *is* a signal, but not that she is out of control. Rather, it's a signal that *she is out of balance, especially with respect to the issue of control.* Trying to control outcomes and emotions by maintaining unreasonably high expectations, driving herself, and manipulating others creates unneeded tension and stress. This leads Jenny to regularly "fill up" by overeating her favorite comfort foods.

Jenny's attempts to maintain control in so many areas of her life create imbalance. Something has to give. She has to *let go* somewhere.

Carla, a shy and reserved thirty-nine-year-old bookkeeper has had difficulty manifesting her desires. Single and alone, she has experienced chronic disappointment in her life, and she feels powerless to change it. After college, she stayed in what she called a "dead-end" job for many years because she "hates change." She hasn't found any type of work that she feels passionate about. She has had few boyfriends over the years and says that her "relationships usually just fizzle out over time."

Carla sees her inability to lose weight as yet another example of her failure in life. She struggles with constant envy of others who appear to have what she desires. Like Jenny, she feels out of control and believes that she *should* be able to control her life and her eating. At times, she tries harder to gain control, but periodically she gives in to the experience of despair. She concludes that she is inadequate, defective in some way, and unlucky and that "others have it all."

Like Jenny, Carla is out of balance with respect to the issue of control. Her life has not felt easy — it has been filled with disappointment, and her infrequent successes have been hard earned. She has experienced much discomfort in life, and she doesn't want any more. So, in an attempt to control her comfort level, she resists change and growth and takes few risks. When she does try new things, she expects an immediate payoff for her efforts and has difficulty surrendering to the slow pace of steady change.

Carla's expectations of herself are low, although they are high regarding weight loss. Her expectations of others are often too high as she looks to them for validation, caretaking, reassurance, and comfort. Trying to constantly control her comfort level by resisting forward movement creates stagnation and frustration and leads to chronic anxiety, depression, and emotional eating. Something has to give. She will have to *let go* of some comfort and take on more risk.

Expending too much effort to control outcomes and maintain a certain comfort level disconnects us from our authentic *feeling self* and robs us of our reserves of vitality and calm. This leads us right back to eating in order to "fill up." Paradoxically, we feel *out of control* because we are trying too hard *to control* our lives. Our *feeling self* is screaming, "*Let go!*"

"I'll Be Happy When…"

Behind our illusions of control lie our beliefs about happiness and contentment. We erroneously believe that these states are contingent upon fulfilling our desires. As emotional eaters, we have the fantasy that *when* we lose the weight, we will be happy. We know that we have plenty of other aspects of our lives to improve, but we believe we will feel much better about ourselves in slimmer bodies. Okay, fair assumption. But as anyone who has reached his or her goals, including weight loss goals, can tell you, soon after you reach a goal, an inner restlessness or emptiness sets in. Reaching a goal is often anticlimactic; it does not produce an enduring sense of joy. Our long-sought-after contentment is fleeting. Happiness now depends on something else we believe we need.

What Then?

I often ask clients this question to help them see that they are putting off to some future time the happiness and contentment that is available to them in each and every moment. The following dialogue with Carla illustrates this point:

> Carla: "I'm miserable in this body. If I just lose twenty to thirty pounds I'll feel much better."
>
> Julie: "I'm sure you will. And once you lose the weight, *what then?*"
>
> Carla: "Then I'll be ready to start dating again."
>
> Julie: "And once you're dating — *what then?*"
>
> Carla: "Hopefully I'll meet the right partner and have a great relationship."
>
> Julie: "That sounds wonderful — and once you have the great relationship with the great guy, *what then?*"
>
> Carla: "Then I'll finally have someone to travel with and see all the places I never get to see."

This dialogue could go on and on. Carla's contentment is constantly on hold. She is *waiting* to feel better about herself, in a slimmer body, to begin dating. She is *waiting* to have a partner to begin traveling. Her happiness is always contingent on achieving the next goal. Any derailment on her path, such as gaining back a little weight, or an unforeseen setback, such as illness or injury, puts her joy even further off.

Carla doesn't have to wait for a slimmer body to feel good about herself. She doesn't have to lose weight to begin dating — plenty of overweight women have partners. And she doesn't have to have a partner to begin seeing the world. She can travel alone or with groups. Carla needs to practice letting go — of the fantasy that her life begins when this or that happens. She must begin to let go of her resistance to being uncomfortable and surrender to the fact that life has lots of manageable discomfort and we can still move forward.

The Drama of Striving

Our lives are constantly filled with the drama of chasing happiness and contentment by either achieving goals and setting new ones or setting goals, failing to achieve them, losing hope, retreating, and at some point starting over. The drama of striving is itself addictive and keeps us regularly distracted. In the midst of the drama, we often fail to stop and ask, "Is there another way?"

The answer is a resounding *yes*! And it's called *letting go*. The truth is that happiness and contentment are always available to you, even during the rough times. They exist at the center of your being and do not depend on anyone or any external circumstance. To be content or not to be content is a choice you make each moment. Doing so involves letting go of whatever gets in the way of your appreciating and surrendering to each moment. You adjust your attitude and stop wasting the preciousness of each moment by longing for it to be different. You bring an attitude of joy to every situation rather than wait for external events to change and produce happiness. Easier said than done, for sure!

Letting Go Begins with Identifying Your Attachments

As humans, we are hardwired to form emotional attachments with each other and other creatures. We begin forming attachments right in the womb. Emotional attachments are necessary for our survival, and they can be a source of tremendous joy throughout our lives.

In our competitive me-focused Western culture, where we define ourselves by whom we know and what and how much we have, it's easy for us to become further attached to material things, conditions, outcomes, states of being, the past, and even our unhealthy behaviors like emotional eating.

These attachments serve us as well. They represent our attempt to find meaning, self-worth, completeness, and wholeness. They represent our attempt to control our comfort level and sense of safety and security in the world. Having lots of money, possessions, or power may give us a feeling of importance as well as security. Holding on to a grudge may provide safety by assuring we do not trust someone or risk anything again.

Our attachment to unhealthy behaviors like complaining and gossiping keeps us safe by taking the focus away from the changes *we* need to make.

Sometimes we are not even aware of an attachment until we are threatened with its loss. An attractive woman may not realize how attached she is to turning heads until the heads aren't turning as much. A businesswoman may not be aware of her attachment to her identity as a successful entrepreneur until her business fails and she files for bankruptcy. Eckhart Tolle, spiritual teacher and author of *A New Earth*, writes:

What Are You Attached to?

THINGS	CONDITIONS	OUTCOMES	UNHEALTHY BEHAVIORS
Power	Comfort	Quick payoff	
Money	Control	Perfection	Overeating/
Identity	Ease	Goals met	Drinking/
Ego	Pleasure	Success	Drug use
Possessions	Achieving	Fairness	Judging
Causes	Striving	Justice	Gossiping
	Struggling		Prejudice
STATES OF BEING	Seeking	**THE PAST**	Negativity
	Searching		Complaining/
Well-known	Drama	Accomplish-	Whining
Well-liked	Freedom	ments	Addictions
Right	Independence	Pleasurable	Denial
Prideful	Space	memories	Magical
Understood/	Safety	Resentments	thinking
Heard	Security	Hurts/Grudges	Codependency
Appreciated		Losses	Caretaking
Respected	**OTHER BEINGS**	Mistakes	Avoidance
Validated		Traumas	Resistance
Approved	Spouse		Defensiveness
Seen/Visible	Partner		
Young/	Children		
Beautiful	Friends		
Athletic	Family		
Smart	Animals		

Many people don't realize until they are on their deathbed and everything external falls away that *no thing* ever had anything to do with who they are. In the proximity of death, the whole concept of ownership stands revealed as ultimately meaningless. In the last moments of their life, they then also realize that while they were looking throughout their lives for a more complete sense of self, what they were really looking for, their Being, had actually always already been there, but had been largely obscured by their identification with things, which ultimately means identification with their mind.

Letting Go Is Scary

You may fear that if you *let go* you won't achieve your goals. You won't get what you want, and you'll lead a frustrated, unfulfilled life. Perhaps you'll feel like a failure and be ashamed. Or maybe you'll become complacent and lazy and your life will be mediocre.

Perhaps you'll be more uncomfortable than you can tolerate. If you *let go* of your resistance to feeling your emotions, you might fall apart and be unable to pull yourself back together. If you take chances socially, you might experience painful rejection. You could risk loss or abandonment if you *let go* and stop your caretaking or people-pleasing behaviors. Perhaps there will be no going back; you will have opened a door you can't close. Maybe you'll be disappointed with the outcome and feel like you wasted time and effort. Letting go would certainly be easier if there were some kind of guarantee that you would get what you want.

Letting go is not necessarily about giving up on your goals, enduring unending discomfort, or ending relationships. It's all about finding balance. We practice letting go of an attachment when it no longer serves our, or someone else's, best interests. If a particular attachment, or the threat of the loss of it, is producing stress, anxiety, or depression, it's creating imbalance, which ultimately leads back to emotional eating.

"How Do I Know When to Hold On and When to Let Go?"

Letting go is about releasing the energy you are wasting by trying so hard to force, push, avoid, or resist "what is" or what you need to do. You relax a bit and allow the flow of your life to carry you in a more harmonious and effortless way. You free yourself to go *with* the flow. You practice accepting life as it unfolds, all the while holding on to your vision of how you would like it to be.

You intuitively balance the act of pushing forward with letting go, surrendering to what is best for you and others in each moment. You remind yourself to enjoy the scenery along the way and work on remaining flexible when you encounter forks, detours, or even blocks in the road. You pay close attention to your emotions and needs and catch and reframe self-defeating thoughts (skills #1 and #2, chapters 2 and 3). You access your Inner Nurturer for soothing and reassurance. This translates into minute-by-minute self-care choices and decisions.

Shakti Gawain, author of the inspirational bestseller *Creative Visualization*, offers a powerful affirmation you can use to help you face fears associated with letting go:

The universe is unfolding perfectly
I don't have to hang on
I can relax and let go
I can go with the flow
I always have everything I need to enjoy my here and now
I have all the love I need within my own heart
I am a lovable and loving person
I am whole in myself
Divine love is guiding me and I am always taken care of
The universe always provides

Of course, feel free to substitute *my Inner Nurturer* or *my highest self* if the term *Divine love* makes you uneasy.

Practice Letting Go in Four Easy Steps

While there are no hard-and-fast rules for learning to let go, you can begin the process of letting go of attachments that no longer serve you or others by taking an honest look at *all* your attachments.

Letting Go Means...

+ accepting and loving yourself *as is*
+ accepting others as they are
+ allowing others the freedom to be themselves
+ not defining yourself by your beauty, money, possessions, or fame
+ sharing what you have with others
+ accepting that you can't always be liked, understood, heard, validated, right, and so on
+ being flexible when things don't go as planned
+ being willing to feel uncomfortable emotions
+ adjusting unrealistic expectations
+ delaying gratification
+ practicing patience
+ releasing perfectionism and accepting "good enough"
+ grieving losses and disappointments
+ forgiving — releasing anger and resentment
+ releasing self-defeating thoughts
+ trying on new, healthier behaviors
+ doing things you don't always feel like doing
+ not personalizing other people's behaviors or comments
+ accepting the pace of change and progress
+ "attracting" rather than "seeking and searching"
+ telling the truth and accepting the consequences
+ going with the flow instead of against it
+ being willing to be uncomfortable

1. Make a list of all your attachments.
   Be sure to include people, animals, things, states of being, conditions, past events, outcomes, and unhealthy behaviors.
2. List the attachments that create imbalance.
   Be honest with yourself. Pick one attachment to begin your practice of letting go. Start small; pick what will be easiest to let go of. Set an intention to work on this issue, and write it down in your journal. For example: "I intend to focus on my attachment to always being comfortable and to relaxing when I'm at home, which results in a cluttered house."

3. Commit to one small change that you can make.

    Write your commitment in your journal: "I commit to hanging up my clothes in the closet rather than piling them on the chair and bed. I will do this immediately after taking them off."

    Then explore your emotions and thoughts regarding letting go. Write down your emotions and thoughts in your journal. What do you fear will happen if you let go? What will you lose or give up? How will you feel? What will you gain? Is it worth the trade-off of being a bit less comfortable? Watch any tendency to get overwhelmed by all that you would like to change. Take it one change at a time. Remind yourself that slow and steady wins the race.

4. Monitor your progress.

    Try putting a check mark on the calendar each time you follow through on your commitment. Or put money in a jar each time you succeed in letting go. When you reach a specified amount, treat yourself to something special. And when you're ready, commit to making another small change.

"*I* Can *Have It All, Just Not All at Once*"

Jenny, the family physician, realized that her attachment to perfection, striving, and having all her goals and desires met *now* was leaving little time for self-care and was creating imbalance. She regularly resorted to using food for excitement and comfort and to wind down from her very long days. In addition, her attachment to being needed translated into loose boundaries, into saying yes when she often wanted and needed to say no. She set an intention to practice letting go in these particular areas.

She decided to resign from two professional boards that she felt were "a waste of time" and committed to reducing her workload by hiring a physician's assistant. These changes felt good and resulted in more time for self-care. Packing healthy snacks and lunches, preparing light dinners, and adding more exercise and sleep to her life immediately translated into weight loss. Jenny realized that she could meet most of her desires and goals *over time* and didn't need to meet them all at once.

Letting go of her attachment to "being included" proved more challenging. Jenny felt anxious when she said no. She committed herself to using soothing Inner Conversations (skill #3, in chapter 4) to validate her need for downtime. She accessed her Inner Nurturer for reassurance that her anxious feelings were actually a sign of progress and that she was taking better care of herself. She began to say no or "Let me think about that and get back to you" more often.

When anxious thoughts surfaced about being left out, Jenny used powerful energizing reframes, such as:

"I need to have quality alone time."
"It may take time for people to adjust to my firm boundaries."
"My family and patients deserve a well-rested caregiver."
"I can say no periodically and will still be invited again."

It came as no surprise to me when, several months into practicing letting go, Jenny reported that she and her husband were expecting a baby boy.

"I Never Realized I Was So Attached to Being Comfortable"

Carla, the bookkeeper, survived her dysfunctional childhood by developing unhealthy behaviors such as avoidance and resistance. These behaviors helped her manage her anxiety and comfort level and resulted in her taking little risk. They also created imbalance and led to a stagnant existence, one filled with anxiety, depression, apathy, inertia, and emotional eating.

Carla set an intention to slowly let go of her resistance to pushing herself out of her comfort zone. She committed to joining a women's exercise class with a twofold purpose: to get in shape and to try to make some new friends. She was considering dropping out after the first session because she found it difficult to keep up with the instructor and didn't see much potential for making new friends with the mostly younger women. Two further areas of attachment were sabotaging Carla's forward movement:

her unrealistic expectations of herself and others; and her desire for an immediate payoff for her efforts.

She realized that in order to honor her intention and commitment, she would have to *let go* of her expectations about getting in shape fast and making new friends. Even though she felt frustrated and impatient, she could tolerate these emotions and some delay in the gratification of her goals.

She committed to practicing soothing Inner Conversations before and after exercise class as needed. She also agreed to write down any negative, hopeless thoughts and replace them with energizing reframes. She replaced "It will take forever to get in shape" with "I am proud of myself for getting to class today; I'm getting stronger each session." And "I'll never make any new friends" became "It takes time to make new friends; I'm on the right track."

Carla stayed with the class for its entire eight-week duration. After the first few weeks, she began to look forward to the class each week, felt a nice sense of community, and had in fact made a few casual acquaintances. When the class ended, she decided to sign up for another eight weeks. Letting go had resulted in more hope and less isolation, depression, and emotional eating. And she had begun to lose weight, without even trying.

CHAPTER SIXTEEN

Practice #3. Fill Your Life with Purpose and Meaning

I lona, a forty-eight-year-old stay-at-home mom, felt a sinking feeling as she dropped her son off at the dormitory of the East Coast college he would be attending. She headed to the nearest restaurant, justifying this to herself by thinking that she'd had too small a breakfast and would need a large, hearty meal to hold her over during the flight back to California. At the airport she bought a romance novel and a large bag of trail mix for the plane ride home. The bag was empty when she exited the plane.

Her husband of twenty-five years greeted her at the airport, and once again she felt a sinking feeling. On the drive home, they stopped for dinner, and Ilona, ravenously hungry, ordered and ate a large, heavy meal. Exhausted from the day, she went right to bed when she arrived home.

She telephoned me the next day, saying, "I'm worried — I think I'm depressed again. I know this is most likely part of an 'empty nest' syndrome, but I can't understand why I'm eating nonstop. I knew the day would come when my youngest son would leave home, and I have a number of interests and hobbies I'd like to pursue. I'm not sure why I'm bingeing and feeling so unmotivated and apathetic."

Ilona, like so many other emotional eaters I work with, learned early in her childhood that it was unsafe to express emotions or needs. She disconnected from her internal world by distracting herself with food and books. She was expected to be a good girl and please others. Her father, like her husband, was a workaholic and rarely home. Her mother was sweet, anxious, and passive.

Ilona didn't feel any real sense of purpose in her life until she had her first child. Raising three boys seemed to give her life the meaning it had been missing. Now that her youngest son was off to college, she felt adrift and her existence seemed devoid of purpose.

Early Nurturance Helps Us Find Purpose

When we are raised in a loving, nourishing, and enriching environment, others notice and encourage our natural abilities, inclinations, strengths, and interests. Our caregivers gently and wisely guide us in pursuing meaningful activities and purpose-filled paths. Whether our interests lead to lifelong vocations or part-time hobbies, we enter adulthood with a clear idea of what we enjoy, what we're good at, and what feels meaningful.

If, instead, we are neglected, raised in an undernourished, chaotic, or traumatizing environment, we will spend our early years *surviving* the neglect, chaos, shame, attack, criticism, and abuse. In our free time we may seek comfort, pleasure, safety, and distraction rather than purpose and meaning.

Fortunate is the child who can, in the midst of neglect or chaos, find meaningful distraction. Usually, such children have a strong, inborn drive and are able to channel it into their studies, sports, musical instruments, art, drama, and the like. They are able to compensate for the lack of nurturance in their environment by driving themselves. They can generally rely on their drive to push them forward.

Other children, often with a more sensitive or passive nature, may not fare so well in discovering meaning and purpose. They may struggle with low frustration tolerance; and without nurturance and proper guidance, they may have difficulty applying themselves throughout their lives. They may feel easily overwhelmed. They may have undetected learning disabilities or attention deficits. While these children may be bright and talented, they often give up on activities they find challenging, quitting too soon to experience the meaning that competency and mastery can bring. Like Ilona, these children often become adults who find themselves in unsatisfying jobs, careers, friendships, and marriages. They find it difficult to make changes because they do not feel inherently driven or motivated. They experience internal resistance to pushing forward.

Purpose Can Be Handed Down

Our life's purpose is sometimes handed down to us from well-intentioned caregivers, with little regard for what we find meaningful. We may be expected to take part in the family business, follow Dad into a military career, or get married and stay at home and raise children. Perhaps we're expected to get an education and pursue a family-approved career in medicine, law, engineering, or accounting. For practicality's sake, we may be discouraged from pursuing our creative interests and passions. It takes courage, motivation, and persistence to break free of these paths later in life and pursue more meaningful activities.

Even though Ilona had been encouraged to go to college, the unspoken message she received from her parents was that she should find a husband and get married. Her father showed little interest in her talent for creative writing and convinced her "not to waste her time." During the course of our work together, Ilona told me:

> Other than raising our sons and being a dutiful wife and daughter, I haven't done much in my life that has felt all that meaningful. Yes, I went to college, but I wasn't a great student. Other kids seemed to know what they wanted to do with their lives. I felt lost and unmotivated. When I met Ted, he had a clear, strong sense of himself and knew he wanted to pursue a career in law. It felt good to be wanted, and being attached to Ted made me feel less lost. Until our first child was born, I worked at a boring secretarial job where I watched the clock all day. I finally felt some meaning and purpose caring for and raising our sons. And truthfully, having children meant I could stay at home and not deal with the whole career thing.

Many Activities Can Be Purposeful

Nothing feels better than waking up and looking forward to the day. Life feels worth living. We feel a sense of fulfillment and satisfaction because our life has purpose and feels meaningful. And it's even better if we feel inspired and passionate about what we're doing.

We can feel purpose and meaning while engaging in many types of activities, including those that

- are routine and provide us with order, satisfaction, comfort, and balance;
- improve our personal lives; and
- improve the lives of others.

Some routine activities are inherently more enjoyable than others. I take a certain pleasure in washing the dishes and cleaning up the sink, but cleaning the shower, while purposeful, leaves me cold. Some activities come easily to us and feel natural and comfortable. In the right mood, I actually enjoy vacuuming because I like moving my body. And some purposeful activities require us to push ourselves out of our comfort zone. This is how I feel sometimes about rewriting chapters.

We become imbalanced when we don't have enough meaningful activity in our lives, and this can lead to eating in an attempt to fill up the emptiness. Likewise, a pursuit of meaningful activities to the exclusion of self-care needs and other responsibilities can equally unbalance us. We need just the right balance.

Does Your Life Feel Purpose Filled?

If your immediate response to this question is no, this lack may help explain your emotional eating. Your life probably contains plenty of purposeful activity, but it's most likely routine and does not feel all that meaningful. Perhaps life feels like one big chore and you're just going through the motions. Maybe you don't feel inspired or passionate about anything.

If your life feels devoid of significance right now, try not to lose hope or faith. It's totally okay to be right where you are. Be compassionate and

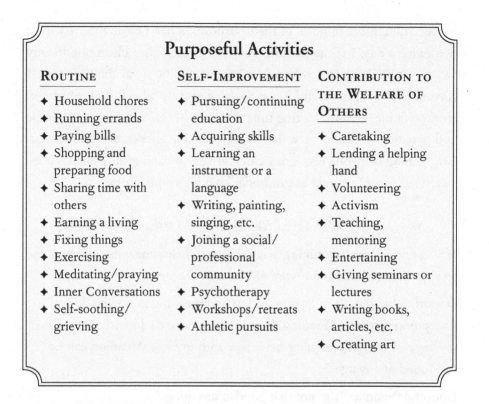

Purposeful Activities

ROUTINE	SELF-IMPROVEMENT	CONTRIBUTION TO THE WELFARE OF OTHERS
✦ Household chores	✦ Pursuing/continuing education	✦ Caretaking
✦ Running errands	✦ Acquiring skills	✦ Lending a helping hand
✦ Paying bills	✦ Learning an instrument or a language	✦ Volunteering
✦ Shopping and preparing food	✦ Writing, painting, singing, etc.	✦ Activism
✦ Sharing time with others	✦ Joining a social/professional community	✦ Teaching, mentoring
✦ Earning a living	✦ Psychotherapy	✦ Entertaining
✦ Fixing things	✦ Workshops/retreats	✦ Giving seminars or lectures
✦ Exercising	✦ Athletic pursuits	✦ Writing books, articles, etc.
✦ Meditating/praying		✦ Creating art
✦ Inner Conversations		
✦ Self-soothing/grieving		

gentle with yourself. Allow yourself to explore the emotions that might be surfacing — they are signaling you that something is out of balance. It will take some time to build more purpose and meaning, but doing so is not impossible.

Four Strategies for Building More Meaning

You *can* fill your life with purpose and meaning; your life can feel significant at any stage or phase. The following four strategies will help you begin the process.

Strategy #1. Adjust Your Daily Attitude

You can add more meaning and joy to your routine activities by focusing on the benefits of certain tasks you perform. Make them more meaningful by becoming more mindful of their purpose. When I clean the kitty litter box twice a day, I focus on how nice it is to provide a clean box for my sweet companions. Recently, when I spent two hours at the tire store, I focused on how purposeful it was to drive on safe wheels. I also brought work with me, and my waiting time felt purposeful. You can offer a smile and a patient attitude to waiters and checkout clerks who serve you. Brightening someone else's day can feel very meaningful. This has been described as an "attitude of gratitude." And it's contagious.

Strategy #2. Catch and Reframe Self-Defeating Thoughts

If you find yourself doubting your ability to bring meaning and purpose to your life, go back and review skill #2, in chapter 3.

Doubtful thought: "I'm just too old to find meaning in my life."

Energizing reframe: "Finding meaning has more to do with my *willingness* to try something new than with my age. Meaning can be found at any age."

Doubtful thought: "I'm not that good at anything."

Energizing reframe: "I have many talents and resources to draw on. I can start by listening to my heart's yearnings."

Doubtful thought: "It's hard to drive myself; I have no support."

Energizing reframe: "I can give myself the support and encouragement I need. As I take a chance, unknown people will show up to support my growth."

Doubtful thought: "I feel empty and depleted. I have little to give."

Energizing reframe: "It's purposeful and meaningful to give *myself* the emotional nurturance I need. As I practice loving and nurturing myself, I feel less empty and depleted. Small acts of self-love have big payoffs."

You may have to act *as if* you believe these reframes until your *feeling self* catches up with your *thinking self*.

Strategy #3. Try Something New

If your personal life feels monotonous, routine, or boring, let your heart guide you in finding more stimulating or joy-filled activities. Is there something you've always wanted to try? You can start with something in your comfort zone, like an online study course or a dance class at a facility with which you are familiar. The important point here is to step out and try something, *anything*, new or different to improve your personal life. Adding more meaningful activities will lead to the nourished, full feeling you're looking for.

Strategy #4. Make a Positive Contribution to Someone Else's Life

While you may feel that all you can handle is to focus on activities that improve *your* personal life, keep in mind that turning your attention to others can help give your life perspective and meaning. Helping others can lift you out of a seemingly purposeless existence. We need soul-nourishing connection with others to feel complete and whole.

Make a list of activities you could take part in that would contribute to the well-being of others. This doesn't have to involve many hours per week; even a couple of hours per month can feel meaningful. Think about what you can offer in terms of time, resources, money, and talent.

Which needs or issues in the world call to you? Which causes feel near and dear to your heart? Maybe you'd like to help others who struggle with challenges you have personally struggled with and conquered. Perhaps you experienced abandonment as a child and it would feel meaningful to volunteer at a group home for children. Maybe volunteering as a Big Sister to a child in need would feel purposeful and create a loving connection. You might want to combine volunteering with one of your interests or hobbies and, for example, become a docent at your local museum, offer your time to a wildlife refuge, or help out during a local election.

Think about who inspires you. Whom would you like to be like? What qualities does this person have that you also have or might cultivate? Perhaps you're inspired by a community leader's tireless efforts to help impoverished souls and clean up the environment. Maybe volunteering to feed the homeless on Thanksgiving Day or participating in a beach cleanup would feel purposeful and inspiring.

Purpose and Meaning Shift as We Grow

Life is ever changing, and as we mature and evolve, different activities take center stage. If we remain open, flexible, and tuned in via our Inner Conversations, our emotions and needs will guide us in finding purpose and meaning at any phase of our lives.

When Ilona was younger, regularly keeping up with friends and family felt purposeful and added significant joy, intimacy, and meaning to her life. As she got older, it felt more purposeful to create quiet, contemplative alone time. While she still kept in touch, she no longer felt the need or desire to stay on top of every detail of everyone's life.

After many years of spending two or more weekends per month volunteering as an environmental activist, Sally no longer felt motivated to go to protests. She still felt passion regarding environmental causes, but it now felt more purposeful to focus her efforts on writing a book on how to care for the planet.

Michele had never found much meaning or passion in her work as a sales manager for a pharmaceutical supply company. Her work served a purpose — it allowed her to put food on the table, pay the rent, and save money to buy a home of her own. She was, however, inspired by nature, and hiking in the mountains most weekends added meaning to her life that was missing during her workweek. She was surprised to find her interest in hiking dwindle when she bought a home, a fixer-upper. While nature would always hold a place in her heart, it now felt more purposeful to devote her time to improving her new abode.

Visiting her husband, Joe, daily in the convalescent hospital felt meaningful to Helen. She arranged her day around visiting him. When Joe passed on, Helen felt displaced. She felt she had lost her purpose in life. Her son suggested she volunteer her time at the hospital, since she had been so comfortable there. After a prolonged period of grieving, Helen decided to give it a try. She was pleased to discover that helping others, many whom were total strangers, inspired her, and once again her days felt purposeful.

Connecting to a Higher Purpose or Calling

At some point in our lives, we all ask questions about the bigger picture: What is the purpose of my life? What am I here on planet Earth to do? What would provide me with a deep sense of satisfaction and meaning?

Your emotional eating may, in part, represent a sense of disconnection from a heartfelt calling or a higher purpose to your life. Each of us has something unique and special to offer this world. Our sense of well-being is greatly enhanced when we contribute to the welfare and enjoyment of others. For some of us, life does not feel personally meaningful *unless* we are making a positive contribution to the lives of others.

Our contribution can be something as simple as feeding a stray cat or as complex as founding and running a global aid organization. The size or type of our contribution truly doesn't matter, only that it comes from the heart.

Whether we discover it early or late in life, we can sense a higher purpose or calling because it has the following features:

- It feels natural.
- It comes easily to us.
- We enjoy it.
- We feel free to be our authentic self.
- It enhances our life.
- It involves a positive contribution to the lives of others.
- We seem to be drawn to it repeatedly.

If your life feels unsatisfying on many levels, and you find you're just getting through each day, you will not have enough energy left over for exploring questions about the bigger picture. Focus your efforts on build-ing your self-care skills (see part 1) and following the body-balancing principles (see part 2) outlined in previous chapters. The desire to find more meaning *will* surface. And it will feel natural to want to share your abundance when you're taking better care of yourself and many of your needs are met.

Honor your resistance — begin stepping out only when you feel ready. But keep in mind that helping others, even in a small way, may pull you out of your self-absorption and isolation, give you an expanded perspective on life, reduce your depression, and curb your emotional eat-ing. The following questions will assist you, when you're ready, in finding your higher purpose or calling:

If you didn't have to work for a living and could do anything you
    wanted to do *to help others*, what might you do?
Which injustices, challenges, or causes in the world make you the
    most angry or sad?
Is there something you feel passionate about that might lead the way
    to a higher purpose?
Is there any message regarding purpose that keeps coming back to
    you that you tend to dismiss because of fear or unfeasibility?
Is there something you would love to try but are afraid to attempt?

As the messages come, *and they will*, think about small steps you could take to align yourself with a potential calling. You don't have to have any particular goal or plan in mind. When you are properly aligned, all kinds of support from the universe will show up. In time you will look back and see how your life unfolded just as it needed to.

"I Never Thought I Could Find Purpose Again in Life"

Ilona had been disconnected from her emotions and needs for so long that she didn't really know herself well. She found it challenging to figure out what she was feeling, and she was afraid to explore for fear she would become more depressed. As she continued to practice self-connection (skill #1, in chapter 2) and form an alliance with her Inner Nurturer, she became aware of four emotions that surfaced regularly: fear, sadness, anger, and grief. During our therapy sessions, Ilona grieved for the child she had been, who received little nurturance and guidance, and for the years of feeling numb and disconnected from herself. She felt sad about her dependency on her husband, Ted, and angry at herself and him for allowing it to occur. She felt afraid that if she expressed her feelings to Ted, he might leave her.

Ilona began to realize that she could allow herself to feel all these emotions without falling apart or eating nonstop. It took time for her to be able to clearly identify her needs and feel safe enough to risk asserting herself. She was slowly defining a separate self and was becoming more comfortable expressing her needs and setting boundaries between herself and others. While Ted did feel a bit threatened by Ilona's more assertive self, he truly wanted the best for her, and he agreed to attend couples therapy to strengthen their marriage.

As her depression began to lift, her apathy, inertia, and overeating diminished. It became easier to stick to limits she set for herself with food and excessive pleasure reading. Ilona now felt ready to explore more purposeful and meaningful pastimes. She decided to step out of her comfort zone and take a class in creative writing at the local college. She discovered that not only did she enjoy writing as much as she had when she was younger but she still had a talent for it. At her professor's suggestion, she submitted one of her essays to a women's magazine. Much to her surprise, it was accepted, and she was later asked to write a monthly column. This was the beginning of a meaningful part-time career writing stories and articles for publications. For the first time in her life, Ilona felt she had found her true calling. No doubt she has touched many lives with the moving stories she has shared about her journey.

CHAPTER SEVENTEEN

Practice #4. Fill Up on Nourishing Connections

Other than during her three-year marriage, Sharon, a forty-four-year-old graphic artist, had been single her entire life. Even though she came from a large, extended family, she had distanced herself from them long ago. Without a partner or children, she often felt invisible at family gatherings. Her parents had both passed away in the previous few years, and Sharon found herself experiencing an overwhelmingly painful and at times paralyzing sense of loneliness. She had few close friends and did not find these connections particularly nourishing. Overeating and oversleeping were Sharon's only ways of coping with chronic depression and despair.

Her thoughts were pessimistic and hopeless: "I'm shy, and I've always been terrible at meeting new people" and "I look awful, and I'm too over-weight to find a life partner." Sharon felt ashamed and labeled herself "pathetic" and "a loser." She cited examples of times when she'd felt so desperate for connection that she had attempted to get to know people too quickly. She believed she had turned them off with her neediness and desperation. She described how, at such times, she might have a nice chat with a stranger in line at the bank and then suggest they meet for lunch. "I feel like a parched plant in the desert, thirsty for any drop of water I can get."

Do loneliness and isolation have anything to do with your emotional eating? Do you lack nourishing relationships in your life, ones where you feel safe, seen, heard, accepted, understood, and loved? Perhaps at times you feel invisible, as if you're living on the outside of the world, looking in. Maybe you long to belong to a community of others with whom you have shared interests and where you experience joy and inclusion. You're not alone.

It's Natural to Want to Connect

We are communal animals, social creatures by nature. We need one another. Throughout human history, the uncomfortable emotion known as loneliness has prompted us to connect with others.

Beyond mere survival, community has always been a source of connection, comfort, support, meaning, and joy. It provides an opportunity to build and practice relational skills. Community offers us an extended family and a larger safety net to rely on.

In our twenty-first-century culture, loneliness is prevalent. In densely populated cities as well as spread-out suburbs, many people feel isolated and cut off from others. In generations past, extended families were the norm, and they represented small communities within larger communities. Divorce was rare, as was the single-person household. Community spirit was alive and well. Neighbors could regularly be seen sitting and chatting on porches, and children played unsupervised in the streets.

Today, the small nuclear family is the norm, and extended family members often live many miles, if not countries, apart. Family members are often estranged by divorce and differing lifestyles. A neighborhood is no longer automatically a community. Families, couples, and singles living in close proximity barely know one another. When we lack the comfort and support of extended family, close friends, and neighborhood communities, our life transitions, such as the birth of a child, the death of a spouse, divorce, an empty nest, or a move to a new location, can result in temporary or prolonged loneliness.

To add insult to injury, modern Western societies promote a sort of rugged individualism that encourages and expects us to focus on actualizing our potential. Many of us have been raised to be more concerned with the competition than the communal good. This heightened self-focus can leave us feeling even more disconnected from others. It's ironic that even though we are better connected than ever before — by the Internet and cell phones — loneliness and social isolation are at an all-time high.

Symptoms of Loneliness

We all feel lonely at times. It's normal to feel lonely when we change jobs, break up with a good friend or lover, or move to a new city. Loneliness is not necessarily the same as being alone. We can feel lonely even when we are with others. And we can be alone and find the experience of solitude enjoyable and rejuvenating. Loneliness becomes problematic when it's chronic or persistent — when we regularly experience a painful sense of separateness and aloneness.

When you feel lonely, you may also feel any of the following:

- Empty
- Invisible
- Unworthy
- Rejected
- Abandoned
- Separate
- Lost
- Detached
- Unlovable
- Hopeless
- Helpless
- Depressed
- Anxious
- Insecure
- Needy
- Apathetic

- Bored
- Disconnected

Loneliness Is Bad for Your Health

Chronic loneliness can seriously compromise your physical and emotional well-being. John Cacioppo, a neuroscientist at the University of Chicago who coauthored, with William Patrick, the book *Loneliness: Human Nature and the Need for Social Connection*, has been studying the effects of loneliness. He found that loneliness can be as harmful to your physical health as smoking or obesity.

As an emotional eater, you may have already noticed that chronic loneliness contributes to depression; overconsumption of high-fat, processed foods and of alcohol; a lack of motivation to exercise; and poor sleep. But you may not be aware that loneliness can increase your blood pressure, risk of stroke, and levels of circulating stress hormones like cortisol. It can disrupt the functioning of your immune system and the regulation of cellular processes and lead to increased wear and tear on and premature aging of your body.

When you're lonely, you're more sensitive, and this can disrupt your ability to enjoy connection that's offered. Because loneliness lowers your self-esteem and confidence, you may feel more threatened by and mistrustful of social situations. You're more likely to negatively interpret events and the behaviors of others and distort social cues. This can make the small social uplifts of everyday life feel less gratifying than they might be if you were less lonely.

Loneliness can impair your ability to respond to stressors as challenges; you're more likely to respond with pessimism and avoidance. This can lead to hopelessness, lack of motivation, and a tendency to endure unpleasant circumstances rather than act effectively to change them.

Connection Is the Key

Chronic loneliness is a symptom and signal that you are disconnected from one or more of the three main sources of soul nourishment and sustenance:

- Self
- Others
- Spirituality

Some level of a positive connection to *all* three sources is essential for good emotional and physical health. The Loneliness Self-Test on the next page will help you identify the source(s) of your disconnection. Understanding the root causes of your loneliness will help you put an end to it and any associated emotional eating.

Connection to Self

In chapter 2, skill #1, I discussed the important developmental skill of self-connection. When we grow up in a nonnourishing, dysfunctional family environment where our emotions and needs are neglected, we learn at an early age to cut ourselves off from our inner world. When emotions surface, we don't know how to handle them. We fail to develop an inner nourishing voice; the inner voice that develops is harsh and self-denigrating. Our thoughts tend to be critical and self-defeating. This leads us to look outside ourselves for comfort, reassurance, and validation.

Our expectations of others tend to be high, and we often find ourselves disappointed. We may be hypersensitive, highly reactive, defensive, demanding, hostile, or needy. When we're disconnected from ourselves, we tend to attract similarly disconnected, nonnourishing souls who have little to give because they too feel empty. They may be overeaters, workaholics, alcoholics, gamblers, sex addicts, narcissists, or codependents.

Our dependency issues, our fear of rejection or abandonment, and our poorly defined personal boundaries lead us to stay too long in nonnourishing, sometimes harmful relationships. The lonelier and more disconnected we feel, the more we look outside ourselves for comfort. Our dissatisfaction with the people we attract may make it more comfortable or safe to withdraw and isolate ourselves rather than venture out and risk more rejection and pain. Of course, this leads to more loneliness and hopelessness, which fuels emotional eating.

Loneliness Self-Test

SELF-CONNECTION

- Are you aware of your emotions and needs and generally able to address them and stay in balance? ❏ Y ❏ N
- Do you regularly talk to yourself in a kind, loving, and supportive way? ❏ Y ❏ N
- Are your thoughts generally positive, uplifting, and hopeful? ❏ Y ❏ N
- Are your personal boundaries clear to you, and are you able to express them easily to others? ❏ Y ❏ N
- Are you able to set limits on yourself and delay gratification in order to achieve your goals? ❏ Y ❏ N
- Do you unconditionally accept yourself and love yourself *as is?* ❏ Y ❏ N

If you answered *yes* to four or more questions, you are doing well with self-connection and may need to focus on developing other sources of emotional nourishment to resolve your loneliness.

If you answered *no* to three or more questions, your loneliness and overeating are due, in part, to a lack of self-connection. Reread part 1 of this book and practice the appropriate missing skills.

CONNECTION TO OTHERS

- Do you have supportive, caring others to talk to who "get" you? ❏ Y ❏ N
- Do you have nourishing others with whom you enjoy spending time? ❏ Y ❏ N
- Do you have fulfilling connections with children or animals? ❏ Y ❏ N
- Is it easy for you to connect to others when you're in social settings? ❏ Y ❏ N
- Do you have good social perception — are you able to see or read others accurately and select kind, emotionally available people as friends? ❏ Y ❏ N
- Are you generally considerate of and sensitive to the feelings and needs of others? ❏ Y ❏ N

If you answered *yes* to four or more questions, you are most likely enjoying one or more nourishing connections. To resolve your loneliness, you may want to increase the amount of time you spend with your current connections or focus on increasing the number of connections. If you are experiencing loneliness and the quality and quantity of time spent with others is sufficient, this may be a sign that you are great at caring for and connecting with others but are lacking a good connection with yourself or a spiritual connection.

If you answered *no* to three or more questions, your loneliness is due, in part, to a lack of fulfilling connections with others. Later in this chapter I discuss how to attract nourishing connections.

Loneliness Self-Test

SPIRITUAL CONNECTION

- Do you regularly carve out time to quiet your mind?   ❏ Y   ❏ N
- Do you make time to connect with something (God, nature, animals) that
  allows you to transcend time and space and gain perspective on life?   ❏ Y   ❏ N
- Do you experience a nurturing connection with your own compassionate
  "highest self"?   ❏ Y   ❏ N
- Do you have a spiritual practice that predictably renews and refreshes you?   ❏ Y   ❏ N
- Do you have a religious practice that nourishes your soul?   ❏ Y   ❏ N

If you answered *yes* to at least one of these questions, you're on the road to developing, or have solidly developed, a spiritual connection. Your loneliness is most likely due to a lack of connection with yourself or nourishing others, or to an insufficient practice of your spiritual connection.

If you answered *no* to all or many of these questions, part of your loneliness is due to the lack of spiritual connection. Later in this chapter I discuss options for building this type of connection.

Make Your House a Home

Without realizing it, you've become lonely because your internal "house" is not a home. Disconnection from your inner source of nourishment has led to a painful, desperate sort of loneliness. Go back and practice the five skills outlined in part 1 of this book. Regularly having Inner Conversations between your *feeling self* and your wise Inner Nurturer will help you stay connected to your emotions and identify your needs. Replacing negative thoughts with powerful, energizing reframes transforms your inner world into the sanctuary it was meant to be. You will be better able to regulate your emotions and behaviors when you know how to self-soothe and grieve losses and disappointments. You will feel safe, entitled, and worthy when you can define your personal boundaries and set appropriate limits. And accepting and loving yourself unconditionally will put an end to the self-rejection and constant shame and inadequacy that leads to isolation and emotional eating.

For now, see if you can *embrace your loneliness*. Accept it and allow it to be, without trying to push it away or distract yourself from it. Perhaps you can give it a name and welcome it without judgment. It is here to teach you something and help you grow.

So Desperate That It Was a Turnoff

Remember Sharon, the forty-four-year-old graphic designer who regularly felt a painful sense of loneliness? I encouraged Sharon to embrace her loneliness and see it as a signal that her *feeling self* felt abandoned by her Inner Nurturer. Showing up in the world with a "please, please feed me" energy was backfiring: it resulted in rejection and more self-judgment, isolation, and overeating. Constantly recycling negative, self-denigrating thoughts after experiencing rejection was lowering her self-esteem.

After a few weeks of practicing self-connection by having Inner Conversations, Sharon reported that the deep, despairing kind of loneliness was lessening. "Even though it's counterintuitive, I realize that whenever I feel that paralyzing sense of loneliness, I need to 'go home' rather than look outside myself for connection."

Sharon decided to explore the possibility of rejoining her extended family, since these were people who knew and loved her, people she had well-established connections with. When she reached out and focused on what she had to offer family members, rather than on what she didn't have in common with them, her extended clan began to reciprocate and reach out to her as well. At times, she had to act as if she felt part of the group when in fact she didn't feel that way, but in general, the positive feelings she got from reconnecting and giving of herself reinforced her continued efforts. She discovered a renewed sense of hope that she could attract more nourishing connections outside the extended family.

If you want to connect with others, you'll need to be emotionally available. This means you cannot be preoccupied with your loneliness, fears, depression, negative thoughts, or problems and challenges. When you're feeling lonely and needy, you're more apt to resort to maladaptive coping patterns like self-absorption and people pleasing. You're also more likely to distort social perceptions and react hypersensitively. These behaviors can push people away and lead to further isolation. This is why it's best to "go home" and practice self-connection until you feel better regulated and balanced.

Connection Is Good for Your Health

Whether we experience loneliness depends on the interplay of our nature and the environment. Some of us have a high need or preference for social connection; others have a low need or desire. Some are more sensitive to the absence of connection than others are. We experience loneliness when the level of social connection we desire is not met. This is our biological prompt to go out and connect.

Whereas too much loneliness is harmful to our health, social connection helps regulate our physiology. When we feel connected, we feel safe. We are less stressed and agitated, and our physical health improves. Social connection lowers levels of frustration, hostility, and depression. We think more clearly and creatively. We are better able to collaborate with others. When we feel connected, we anticipate and often experience positive emotions that provide immediate psychological uplift. We are happier and enjoy life more.

Researchers have identified the hormone oxytocin, which emanates from the pituitary gland, as a feel-good chemical. Oxytocin encourages bonding and social connection. First associated with breast-feeding, oxytocin is now known to be released into the bloodstream in response to soothing and connecting behaviors such as hugs, back rubs, lovemaking, and even thumb sucking. Eating also stimulates the release of this chemical of calm, as does drinking moderate amounts of alcohol, and this explains in part why these behaviors are self-soothing. Oxytocin lowers levels of stress hormones and blood pressure and increases our tolerance for pain. It boosts our mood and can result in more positive and adaptive behavior, leading to greater opportunities for social connection.

Attracting Nourishing Others

Breaking free from the grip of loneliness and attracting new connections or reconnecting with previously made contacts may seem like an impossible task. The neglect, abuse, or trauma you experienced as a child robbed you of the opportunity to build adequate self-care and social skills, and perhaps you don't feel equipped to attract kind, nurturing others. As you learn and practice the self-care skills outlined in part 1 of this book, keep in mind that everything you need in order to feel whole is already inside you. You were born whole. The key is to respond to others from your wholeness rather than from your perceived brokenness or "I need"-ness. When you slip back into perceiving yourself as needing something outside yourself, try using positive affirmations to remind you of your wholeness:

"I already have everything I need inside myself to feel whole."
"I am whole and complete."
"I do not need anyone or anything to complete me."
"I am full of inner love; I have much to offer others."
"I effortlessly attract nourishing others by sharing my wholeness."

To better understand the concept that you are already whole, think about the times when you have either been in love or had a full, nourished feeling after spending time with another being or in nature. You headed out into the world feeling joyful and expansive, better able to give of yourself and spread good cheer. These feeling states, associated with wholeness and fullness, were already inside you. You were better able to access them in the presence of a loving or nourishing connection. Your perceived *hole* was filled up with your own *wholeness*.

As you regularly practice a loving, supportive connection with yourself, you begin, perhaps for the first time, to experience your wholeness. The strong need to get something from others subsides; and as you continue to nourish yourself internally, you more often experience a desire to give or share your bounty. A better-self-connected you will naturally and effortlessly attract kind, loving, self-connected others. It will be easier to spot emotionally healthy adults who can nourish, appreciate, and respect you.

"It's Easier Than I Expected"

After months of positive connections with extended family members, Sharon felt willing to take on more challenges. She decided to take a meditation class at a local spiritual center, hoping to combine her interest in Eastern spirituality with her desire to make new connections.

> I don't feel as lonely or needy for connection as I did before, and I can see how differently people are relating to me. It feels easier to connect now — I seem to attract people just by being myself. I don't have to try so hard. And when I get home, I'm not heading straight for the refrigerator!
>
> A group of women around my age invited me to join them for coffee after class on Saturday mornings. It's the highlight of my week. I don't know whether any of them will become close friends, but I'm not concerned about that. I'm just focusing on increasing positive connections in my life and getting clear on which traits or qualities I'm looking for in a friend.

Ten Strategies for Attracting Soul-Nourishing Connections

While there is no simple formula for attracting nurturing others into your life, here are several strategies you can employ to increase the odds.

STRATEGY #1. FOCUS ON INCREASING YOUR EXPERIENCE OF CONNECTION

Rather than attempting to go out and find new friends or a love interest immediately, start small by focusing on casual, positive connections. Smile at the bank teller, compliment the grocery clerk, give someone directions, or pet a friendly dog and say hello to its guardian. Connections that involve giving or helping others elicit positive physiological sensations called the "helper's high." These positive feelings are motivating and can help you push past the passivity, self-absorption, and withdrawal associated with loneliness. The simple act of smiling can improve your mood and connect you briefly to another. Notice the good feelings you get from simple acts of kindness.

STRATEGY #2. BOOST OXYTOCIN BY TOUCHING AND BEING TOUCHED

Take every possible opportunity to appropriately touch others: give someone a hug, neck rub, or back rub, pat someone on the back, or touch someone's hand lightly. Hug and hold your furry friends. If it's within your budget, get a regular massage. The mood boost can result in positive feelings and more adaptive behavior leading to greater opportunities for social connection.

STRATEGY #3. ENVISION THE TYPE OF PERSON YOU WOULD LIKE TO ATTRACT AS A FRIEND

What qualities or traits are you looking for? Get clear on what is most important to you by writing your vision in your journal. Sharon wrote:

I'd like to meet a female friend, around my age, who is

- kind and caring;
- emotionally open;
- nonjudgmental;
- capable of taking an interest in my welfare;
- playful and humorous;
- a professional;
- interested in some of the things I'm interested in; and
- open to spirituality.

Try being proactive when socializing, and make contact with people who have the traits you are looking for. Don't just take those who take you.

STRATEGY #4. INCREASE YOUR ODDS OF CONNECTION

Become better connected by taking part in new activities where you will have repeated contact with others and an opportunity to interact. This allows you to get to know people and determine if they meet the criteria on your vision list. Select activities you enjoy; it's easier to connect with others when you have similar interests and feel engaged. These activities might include the following:

- An interactive cooking or language class
- A book club
- A walking or hiking group
- A fine-dining or theater group
- A volunteer program

STRATEGY #5. ADJUST YOUR EXPECTATIONS

Rather than expecting to make a new friend, expect to increase your practice of social connection and perception skills. It may take several attempts at different social activities over an extended period before you find a comfortable fit with others or make a new friend. You can stay positive by viewing every attempt at connection as progress in skill building. And this includes building the important skill of delaying gratification.

STRATEGY #6. FOCUS ON COMMONALITIES
RATHER THAN DIFFERENCES

When you find yourself feeling uncomfortable and lonely around others, it's natural to want to withdraw and easy to conclude that you have nothing in common. Try a different approach: *look for the similarities.* This will help you feel more comfortable, and you can even try reaching out by commenting on the similarities:

"I like your hat; I'm a hat lover myself."
"I heard you say you're fond of animals; me too."

"I see we've both brought a homemade dessert to this potluck.
Do you enjoy baking?"
"What you said about the story line of the book really resonated
with me. Overall, did you enjoy the book?"

We can almost always find something we have in common with others.
We can connect more easily when we focus on our similarities. We may
not make a lifelong friend, but we will certainly build connections and
goodwill.

Strategy #7. Practice Kind, Available, Generous Behavior

When you're with new people, take a genuine interest in them. Kind-
ness and emotional availability are very attractive; self-absorption is not.
If you notice there's no reciprocity of interest and care, take note of this.
This person may not be someone you want to get to know further.

Strategy #8. Gravitate toward the Warmth

Move toward people who are kind and welcoming. Even though they
may not become your new best friends, the experience of warmth and
acceptance will be the positive reinforcement needed to motivate you to
keep getting out socially.

Strategy #9. Break Old Patterns

If, in the past, you've attracted or accepted as friends certain nonnourishing types, pay attention to how you feel in your body when you're
around these types. Your body is your best guide to what does or doesn't
feel comfortable. Sharon noticed that she felt agitated and invisible around
people who

- talk endlessly about themselves;
- show little or no interest in others;
- are judgmental or shaming;
- engage in a lot of drama; or
- are highly reactive.

STRATEGY #10. DON'T PERSONALIZE OTHER PEOPLE'S STUFF

If you give someone a warm hello or compliment him and get a grouchy or dismissive response, remind yourself that his reaction or behavior has nothing to do with you. Similarly, if you experience social rejection from unfriendly folks, tell yourself, "How sad — these people don't allow themselves to get to know new people. It's their loss." Then see if you can move on.

Watch any tendency to focus on the negativity by recycling negative, angry, or hopeless thoughts. Don't waste time and energy focusing on what doesn't feel good — it just attracts more of the same to you. Remind yourself that there are many more fish in the sea. Continue with your mission to attract kind, available energy.

Spiritual Connection

The third main source of soul nourishment and sustenance is spiritual connection. Spiritual awareness or "awakening" involves an expansion of consciousness beyond our material, day-to-day concerns. How do you know if your emotional eating represents a hunger or yearning for spiritual connection and nourishment? The lack of a spiritual connection may be experienced as a restlessness or sense of unease, discontent, or dissatisfaction with life, even at times when life seems relatively fulfilling. We're often not ready for this type of growth work until we experience some sort of opening.

For the emotional eater who struggles to cope from day to day, spirituality may be the farthest thing from her mind. And yet suffering the pain of disconnection on many levels, over and over again, may trigger the opening needed to search for a nurturing spiritual connection. Even a budding connection can be the light her soul needs in order to keep on going.

For the emotional eater whose life feels relatively full, it may be a periodic emptiness, restlessness, or sense that nothing brings everlasting joy that leads to a search for nourishment beyond the physical.

Spiritual connection involves letting go of our small earthly self and surrendering to something seemingly unknown. Paradoxically, we need to have a fairly solid sense of self to fully surrender. When we don't feel solid, surrender can feel like an unwanted loss of control or a sense of fragmentation or nonexistence. As we become more secure, we begin to see that with spiritual awakening, we *gain* a soul-enhancing, transcendent connection rather than lose our sense of control and sense of self.

Finding the Right Path

Most of us were exposed to some sort of organized religious practice in childhood. For some, religious practice is nourishing from the start and naturally satisfies the need for spiritual connection. Others find occasional spiritual fulfillment by participating in religious traditions on holidays and special occasions. If you currently have no defined spiritual practice and would like to begin the search for one, consider the following options.

1. Explore Spiritual Traditions or Philosophies That Interest You

Perhaps you have always been intrigued by Zen Buddhism or Hindu philosophy. Maybe you've longed to participate in African drumming. Take a class, attend a gathering, or buy a book and begin to explore a new path of interest.

2. Take a Class in Meditation

Try any technique that calls to you. Check for classes offered by spiritual or meditation centers, churches, temples, ashrams, and even adult schools and university extensions.

3. Revisit Your Birth Religion

If this calls to you, go back as an adult with an open mind and explore your birth religion. Perhaps certain practices in your religion appeal to you more than others do. If you were born Christian, perhaps a larger church with a gospel choir would be more attractive than the small church of your youth. If you were born Jewish, you may want to explore Kabbalah, or mystical Judaism. Let your inclinations guide you.

4. PRACTICE YOGA REGULARLY

Any type of yoga will do. I discuss yoga in practice #1, in chapter 14.

5. SPEND TIME COMMUNING WITH NATURE

Carve out time regularly for a walk along the ocean, river, or stream's edge, a walk or hike in the mountains or woods, or a stroll in a park or meadow. Consciously choose to quiet your mind in nature as you take in the sights and sounds. I've always found that my weekly walk along the beach puts life in perspective. It's a humbling, spiritual experience; the ocean is vast, awe inspiring, and incredibly calming to me.

6. SPEND QUALITY TIME WITH ANIMALS

Animals live in the present moment, and they offer unconditional love. Connection to animals can open up unknown parts of yourself. If you aren't currently an animal guardian, consider fostering or adopting an animal or volunteering at a shelter or wildlife sanctuary. A nourishing soul connection to a furry companion may be just the right form of spirituality for you.

7. CONNECT WITH YOUR HIGHER SELF REGULARLY

Your higher self is the wise, loving, expansive advisor that exists within you and communicates to you through intuition, feeling states, insight, epiphanies, and revelations. Contact your higher self by quieting your mind and imagining this part of yourself. You might picture it as a beautiful radiant light or ethereal being. Ask your higher self to assist you in making this connection. Ask for insight and wisdom. As you continue to practice your connection with this part of yourself, it can become the main source of nourishing guidance in your life.

"I Never Saw Myself as a Spiritual Person"

Already feeling somewhat comfortable with her new acquaintances from the spiritual center, Sharon decided to push herself a bit further.

> One of the ladies from my meditation class invited me to a Buddhist "day of retreat" for beginners. Although I was hesitant, I was also curious. But something happened when we were doing this chanting exercise. I felt a sense of peace and well-being come over me that I had never felt before. It stayed with me for the entire day. I'm not sure what I would call it, but I knew I wanted to experience it again. And when I got home I didn't feel like bingeing as I often do when I push myself to try something new. It's all very exciting.

Opening yourself up to spiritual connection requires you to keep an open mind and release any preconceived notions you may have. Regardless of your belief system, regular practices that increase this type of connection will help alleviate and resolve your loneliness and associated emotional eating.

CHAPTER EIGHTEEN

Practice #5. Practice Gratitude

As I sat in the waiting room of my dermatologist's office, I felt sorry for myself. This was the second time in six months that a pimple wouldn't go away and turned out to be skin cancer. Six months earlier, I'd had a recurrence of a previously removed skin cancer. I was one of the *lucky* 1 percent whose cancers recur after the very specialized surgery. Another surgery and one more scar on my face. Why, I wondered, couldn't these growths occur someplace less conspicuous on my body, *like the bottom of my feet!* And why me? After all, I was never really a sun worshiper, although I did have my fair share of sunburns as a child.

Then it dawned on me. I truly had a lot to be grateful for. For one thing, this was not the scary skin cancer called melanoma that could spread throughout the body. Mine was a very slow-growing type, and it didn't require chemotherapy. I was fortunate to be living in a city with great medical care and well-trained physicians. My dermatologist and her staff were kind, compassionate, and supportive. I had medical insurance that covered a good part of the expense. And of course, thank God for scar-minimizing creams, makeup, and dermal fillers that could, at least temporarily, make scars and dents nearly invisible!

Gratitude — it's a powerful tool, an "in the moment" mindfulness practice that can open your heart and shift your perspective. It connects you more deeply to yourself, others, and your Source. The practice of gratitude isn't a way of glossing over or denying life's disappointments and challenges; rather it's a means of freeing yourself from a constant preoccupation with the negative aspects of your life. You are living in *this* moment, present to whatever you're experiencing, grateful for the ever-unfolding journey called life.

If you're depressed and anxious, you're probably not thinking much about gratitude. After all, what's there to be grateful for when you hate your body, feel anxious or worried all the time, are disappointed in your accomplishments, are dissatisfied with your closest relationships, or can't stop overeating? It's hard to feel grateful when you wish you had someone else's life or, worse, that you were no longer alive. As counterintuitive as it may sound, these are the times when you can benefit the most from the practice of gratitude.

The Three Types of Gratitude

When we were young, most of us learned to practice gratitude as if it were a chore. We were prodded to say thank you regularly and encouraged to write notes of appreciation for gifts received. And some of us were required to recite rote prayers of gratitude before meals and at bedtime.

For most of us, as we matured, our periodic heartfelt expressions of gratitude replaced the dutiful, ritualized practices of our youth. Few of us, however, were ever exposed to the concept that a regular and conscious practice of gratitude could be a means to achieving higher states of consciousness and deeper levels of connection and joy.

The practice of gratitude can be broken down into three types. Each type has its benefits; each prepares you for the next type, which is more expansive and transformative than the previous one.

Type 1. Lip-Service Gratitude

If you were asked to make a list of the things you're grateful for, what would it include? Most likely, you would list important relationships, life circumstances, and possessions, such as:

- your health
- your family and friends and their health
- your significant other
- food on your table
- a secure job
- a comfortable place to call home
- your car
- your companion animals
- your connection to a higher power or your "Source"

In truth, most of us have a tendency to take for granted the items on our lists and to focus on what *isn't* working in our lives. I call this most basic type of gratitude "lip-service gratitude" because we usually express and experience it for only a moment and then go back to focusing on our problems. We generally express this type of gratitude for one of four reasons:

1. To boost our spirits when we're feeling down, negative, or just plain blah — "It's really not that bad; at least I have a roof over my head."
2. To pump up a weak ego by flaunting our good — "I'm so blessed to have such a successful business and so many wonderful clients."
3. To highlight our awareness of our good fortune so that we don't appear ungrateful — "I know that I'm fortunate to be married to a wonderful man like Jim."
4. To let others know that even though we're complaining, *we know* that we don't really have it all that bad — "I know that, relative to others, I have it pretty good."

There's nothing wrong with this type of gratitude. It's a valuable practice because it reminds you of your priorities and can temporarily lift you up when you're down. It takes you out of your never-ending focus on good and bad, right and wrong, and allows you to simply fill up on the good that is ever present — the good that we all tend to take for granted. The problem is that it doesn't create deeper change in you, and it isn't particularly effective in combating the spiritual depletion and inner emptiness that drive emotional eating.

Type 2. Attitude Gratitude

Unlike type 1 gratitude, the second type is not just a temporary state we enter when things are going well or as compensation when we feel down and dissatisfied with our situation. Type 2 gratitude represents a more permanent underlying shift in attitude. Your feeling of gratitude goes beyond your life circumstances and possessions and is actually independent of outcomes. You're grateful for all your experiences, positive and negative, and you see them as part of the journey called life. You've come to realize that life has constant ups and downs and that there's always much to be grateful for. If you were to make a list of things you're grateful for while experiencing this type of gratitude, your list might include everything on the previous list, plus things such as:

- your mistakes and failures
- your trials and tribulations (including your relationship with food)
- your obstacles
- your phenomenal physical body
- your very existence
- freedom, as you know it
- the planet and the universe

As with type 1 gratitude, you may find that you shift in and out of this attitude, but with practice it can become the state of mind you live in most of the time. Type 2 gratitude can offer warp-speed mind, body, and spirit healing.

Stop for a moment and reflect on some of the near-miraculous activities taking place outside your conscious mind as you read this paragraph. Some examples:

- Your intestines are converting the food you recently ate into energy.
- Your heart is beating and circulating blood throughout your system.
- Your brain is processing and absorbing the information on this page.
- Your eyes are absorbing reflected light, which assists you in reading this page.

Pretty incredible, if you ask me!

Focusing on your most basic blessings offers, at a minimum, many benefits. On a purely physical level, it's calming and reduces stress. It can temporarily lower anxiety and lift depression by quieting your mind and interrupting self-defeating thoughts and deeply ingrained pessimism and hopelessness. And shifting to a more appreciative outlook opens you up to new possibilities and hope.

As you expand your practice of gratitude by acknowledging and appreciating those around you, a nourishing sense of connection permeates all your activities and encounters. An attitude of gratitude is attractive and contagious. You don't have to like everything about your friends, family members, or colleagues to appreciate their contribution to your life or the common good. Gratitude can act as a lens that softens disappointments and painful experiences and opens you up for further emotional healing. And by focusing you on the good that another person brings into your life, gratitude helps you adjust your expectations.

By consistently practicing type 2 gratitude, you will no longer be thrown off balance by trials and tribulations, because you will expect them. And even though they involve discomfort, you will view them as positive growth experiences. As you continue to let go of your attachment to the idea that things must go your way, it will become clear that happiness is a decision you *can* make each moment.

In the midst of pain and suffering, you notice that love and joy are all around, and you know that it is yours for the taking. To some this may sound crazy — how can I feel joy when I'm in physical or emotional pain? How can I feel love when I'm all alone? The answer lies in the fact that when you are no longer attached to specific outcomes, you are free to see the silver lining in everything. When you're hospitalized with chest pain, you're grateful for the hospital, doctors, and helpful staff and for the loud wake-up call about your self-care. When your husband of ten years tells you he's leaving you for his secretary, you're grateful that someone who no longer wants to be with you is on his way out. You're also grateful for the next leg of your journey, as uncertain and uncomfortable as it may be. You are able to remind yourself that while you are responsible for providing what you believe to be missing in your life, you are never truly alone. You live in an abundant universe full of unforeseen helpers.

You experience joy when you observe a couple in love, even though you are single and at times lonely. Rather than recycle a thought like "They have love and I don't," you are more apt to think, "How wonderful it is to see love — that's joyous and I can share in that." When your best friend tells you she is pregnant and *your* clock is ticking loudly, you experience an intense joy that overshadows *your* longing to be a mother. You know the miracle of life is once again unfolding, and for this you are grateful.

At this point, you may be thinking, "Hey, that sounds great, but I'm not Mother Teresa." True, but you don't have to aspire to be another Mother Teresa to make the choice to enjoy the benefits of an attitude of gratitude.

Type 3. I Am Gratitude

The third type of gratitude represents a continuous state of gratefulness, one that you don't shift into or out of. Rather than practicing gratitude, you live it, *all the time*. With this type of gratitude, you transcend your daily preoccupation with your small self and experience a sense of oneness with everything. Your life is about selfless service and giving back, because all your needs are met.

Some might call this a mystical state, reserved for the likes of avatars such as the Buddha, Jesus Christ, Mother Teresa, and the Dalai Lama. Most of us mere mortals won't experience this type of gratitude completely in our lifetimes, but if we're practicing type 2 gratitude, we may get glimpses of the mystical experiences this type of gratitude can reveal.

You can begin to develop type 3 gratitude, a state of ecstatic appreciation, by regularly acknowledging, and really feeling, gratitude for things that have nothing to do with you or your pleasure. For example, when you turn on the nightly news, you might feel grateful for the heroic efforts of tireless firefighters and relief workers around the globe. I experienced a deep sense of this type of gratitude while watching the Chilean miners being pulled up, one by one, from miles beneath the earth. It was truly miraculous.

Strengthening Your Gratitude Muscle

Here are some tips for pumping up your gratitude muscle:

1. Make a list of everything you are grateful for today.
2. Add to your list things you take for granted that you didn't include on your original list. You might add running water, easily available food, paved roads, and so on. Stop for a moment and reflect on what it takes to bring these things into your life.
3. Throughout the day, practice consciously noticing things for which you are grateful. Take note that you easily found a convenient parking space and that the store manager was helpful and friendly. Make it a point to practice gratitude every time you eat something. Reflect on how the food got to your table and how fortunate you are to have easy access to food and to have a body capable of utilizing it.
4. Practice gratitude even when you don't feel like it. When you deal with a difficult client or coworker, or when you experience some sort of rejection or disappointment, look for the growth opportunity and lesson to be grateful for.

5. Actively look for opportunities to practice gratefulness. Saying "thank you" and expressing heartfelt appreciation as often as possible helps build your gratitude muscle.

6. Begin each day with a gratitude prayer. Express your appreciation, either silently or aloud, for all your blessings and trials. This doesn't have to take long, and it's a great way to start the day, connecting to and from your heart.

Gratitude Reconnects You

Disconnection from your *feeling self*, your Inner Nurturer, your physical body, other people, your highest purpose, and your Source is the root cause of your emotional eating and dissatisfaction. A regular practice of gratitude will help you reconnect, and it doesn't matter what level you're starting at. At its most basic level, gratitude is a gift you give yourself. It's a way of reconnecting first to your own heart and then to everyone and everything else.

Afterword

At this point, you may be wondering, "How long will it take to give my emotional eating the boot?" Perhaps you'd like to know the success rate of this approach and how quickly you can expect to lose weight. No doubt, you've grown accustomed to diet programs promising results within a short time frame, and you'd love some sort of guarantee.

While I can't promise you a certain amount of weight loss within a particular time frame, I can tell you that the approach I've outlined in this book offers you a way out of dieting and a once-and-for-all resolution to your emotional eating. Restrictive dieting has allowed you to periodically put on the brakes, gain a sense of control, and lose some weight, but it hasn't really worked well for you. The truth is, dieting hasn't led to a permanent solution. Rather, it has left you emotionally, physically, and spiritually depleted. The constant focus on food, weight loss, and body image have crowded out joy and vitality and replaced them with vigilance, anxiety, and frustration.

The causes that underlie your overeating or imbalanced eating and weight gain have most likely existed for a very long time. It will take some time to resolve them. This approach will require a shift in your thinking, a longer-term perspective, and a loving commitment to yourself. It's best if you can shift your focus to *gaining* skills and practices rather than to *losing* weight. Over time, the weight will come off and stay off. And you'll find, like everyone else who has lost weight with this approach, that the weight loss part feels somewhat effortless.

For some, like Mary, skill building and weight loss have occurred fairly quickly:

It's truly amazing — I've lost forty pounds this year and never once felt like I was on a diet. The only way I've lost that much weight in the past was by strict dieting and overexercising. I'm a real foodie — I love this eating plan and find it very easy to follow. And my health is better than it's ever been. But most important, I've gained the skills I need to comfort myself when I'm having a rough time. I've always looked outside myself, to food, my husband, or my sisters, for soothing, and it's never felt like enough. Now I know how to turn inward for the support I need, and food just doesn't have the same appeal.

For others, like Anne, the process is slower:

When I can be kind, gentle, and patient with myself, I do better with eating and exercise. I've lost some weight, but the perfectionistic voice in my head tells me it's never enough. If I overeat at a meal, gain back a pound, or have any setback, such as an injury, I quickly slip back into negative, hopeless thinking. But it's easier now for me to catch myself doing this, reframe my thoughts, and have my Inner Nurturer remind me that this is a journey full of ups and downs. For the first time in my life, I'm feeling hopeful about all of this.

Emotional eating has served many purposes in your life. It has helped you cope, and it's truly a blessing in disguise: it highlights a disconnection that has been robbing years from your life. Letting go of long-standing patterns of coping and ways of viewing yourself that no longer serve you is not without challenge. Deep-seated emotions and deeply entrenched self-defeating thoughts are bound to surface. Self-doubt may be a regular visitor. Your old pain will surely demand attention. Setbacks can and will occur. At times you may feel resistant to doing the work required.

Your challenge is this: Do not give up or lose hope. Refer to this book every day until the applicable skills, principles, and practices become second nature to you. Stay the course. Get professional assistance if you need it. You *will* put an end to your emotional eating. I believe in you, and now you must believe in yourself.

Thank you for allowing me to share your journey. I wish you all the best. Let me know how it goes.

Acknowledgments

This book, years in the making, could not have been accomplished without the generous help and support of many. My heartfelt appreciation and deepest gratitude to:

My clients and every person who has attended the Twelve-Week Emotional Eating Recovery Program, my seminars, my workshops, and my emotional-eating support groups over the past twenty-two years. You have been my greatest teachers, helping me to clarify my thinking and teaching methods. Thank you for allowing me to share your journeys of recovery and for having the courage to place your trust in me. You constantly challenge and inspire me to be my best.

Sara R. Beck, for reading, editing, rereading, and reediting the manuscript, at just the right time, and for her continuous and enthusiastic encouragement and support.

Dr. Len Felder, who took the time to carefully critique and reread the book proposal and manuscript, and who offered insightful commentary and caring support.

Dr. Janice Stanger, for reading and editing the manuscript, for offering her invaluable knowledge and assistance regarding plant-based nutrition, and for her continued support of this book.

Dr. Hyla Cass, who, despite her busy schedule, enthusiastically agreed to edit the manuscript and provide astute commentary regarding body and brain imbalances.

Holly Schoellhammer, for hashing out chapter headings during our stair workouts, for her thoughtful attention to the manuscript, and for her wonderful encouragement throughout the entire process.

Dr. David Jimenez, for his kindness and ongoing support of this project, especially during our lunch and dinner meetings.

Paul Levine, my agent, for catching the vision of this project immediately, trusting his instincts, and shepherding this book to just the right publisher.

Marc Allen, my New World Library publisher, for catching the vision as well and for his enthusiastic support of this project.

The wonderful and supportive staff at New World Library: Georgia Hughes, my editor, for her patience and incredible talent in managing the entire editorial process and shaping this book into its current form; Kristen Cashman, managing editor, for her patience and sharp editorial savvy and for cheerfully keeping me on track with editorial details; Jonathan Wichmann, assistant editor, for his kind and warm support; Bonita Hurd, copy editor, for her ever-so-gentle and considerate manner and superb copy editing skills; and Tracy Cunningham, for her talent and creativity in designing the book's cover.

The many talented and gifted researchers and authors who have studied and written about overeating, weight loss, child development, trauma, and recovery and who have informed my life's work.

The physicians, nutritionists, and authors who are knowledgeable about plant-based nutrition and who work so hard to ensure the health and safety of all of the earth's creatures.

The teachers, therapists, gurus, and authors, too numerous to name, who greatly inspired me, contributed to my evolution as a therapist, and awakened and nurtured my spirituality.

My supportive and encouraging friends and spiritual community at the Siddha Yoga Meditation Center.

My mother, for her constant love, support, and belief in me. Our relationship has offered me the greatest opportunity for learning about love, healing, compassion, and forgiveness.

My Source, who is ever present, gracing me daily with love, light, and divine guidance. And my angel Maurine, whom I can't touch but can always feel.

Notes

Chapter One: When Overeating Is Driven by Emotional Hunger

Page 9 *"toxic shame: the feeling of being flawed"*: J. Bradshaw, *Homecoming: Reclaiming and Championing Your Inner Child* (New York: Bantam, 1990), p. 47.

Chapter Two: Skill #1

Page 37 *Laurel Mellin, author*: L. Mellin, *The Solution: 6 Winning Ways to Permanent Weight Loss* (New York: HarperCollins, 1997), p. 177.

Chapter Three: Skill #2

Page 46 *Aaron T. Beck, MD, author*: A. Beck, *Cognitive Therapy and the Emotional Disorders* (New York: International Universities Press, 1976).

Chapter Five: Skill #4

Page 102 *M. Scott Peck, MD, author*: M. S. Peck, *The Road Less Traveled* (1978, repr: New York: Simon and Schuster, 2003), p. 19.
Page 103 *Peck suggests*: Ibid., p. 22.

Chapter Six: Skill #5

Page 118 *Albert Ellis, PhD, founder*: A. Ellis and M. Powers, *The Secret of Overcoming Verbal Abuse* (North Hollywood, CA: Wilshire, 2000), p. 121.
Page 127 *Unrealistic expectations lead to*: K. Horney, *Neurosis and Human Growth* (New York: W. W. Norton, 1950), pp. 65–66.

Page 137 *I first learned of mirror work*: S. Orbach, *Fat Is a Feminist Issue* (New York: Paddington Press, 1978), p. 87.

Chapter Seven: When Overeating Is Driven by Body Imbalance

Page 143 *Americans spend over $65 billion*: Marketdata Enterprises, *The U.S. Weight Loss and Diet Control Market Biennial Study*, May 2011, www.marketdataenterprises.com /DietMarket2011TOC.pdf.

Page 143 *research demonstrates that 98 percent of all dieters*: National Institutes of Health, "Methods for Voluntary Weight Loss and Control" (Technology Assessment Conference Statement), *Annals of Internal Medicine* 116 (1992): 942–49.

Page 146 *According to David A. Kessler, MD*: D. A. Kessler, *The End of Overeating* (New York: Rodale, 2009), p. 145.

Chapter Eight: Principle #1

Page 160 *Doug J. Lisle, PhD, and Alan Goldhamer, DC*: D. J. Lisle and A. Goldhamer, *The Pleasure Trap* (Summertown, TN: Healthy Living Publications, 2003), pp. 69, 64.

Page 165 *The Institute of Medicine . . . suggests*: Institute of Medicine, *Food and Nutrition Board, Dietary Reference Intakes: Water, Potassium, Sodium, Chloride, and Sulfate* (Washington, DC: National Academies Press, 2004).

Chapter Nine: Principle #2

Page 173 *According to the U.S. Food and Nutrition Board*: Institute of Medicine, Food and Nutrition Board, *Dietary Reference Intakes for Energy, Carbohydrate, Fiber, Fat, Fatty Acids, Cholesterol, Protein, and Amino Acids* (Washington, DC: National Academies Press, 2005), p. 589.

Page 174 *A study published in 2004*: A. Astrup, "Atkins and Other Low-Carb Diets: Hoax or an Effective Tool for Weight Loss," *Lancet* 364 (2004): 898. See also G. D. Foster et al., "A Randomized Trial of a Low-Carbohydrate Diet for Obesity," *New England Journal of Medicine* 348, no. 21 (2003): 2087; L. Stern et al., "The Effects of Low Carbohydrate versus Conventional Weight Loss Diets in Severely Obese Adults," *Annals of Internal Medicine* 140, no. 10 (May 18, 2004): 784.

Page 174 *In 2005, the* Journal of the American Medical Association: M. L. Dansinger et al., "Comparison of the Atkins, Ornish, Weight-Watchers, and Zone Diets for Weight Loss and Heart Disease Risk Reduction: A Randomized Trial," *Journal of the American Medical Association* 293, no. 1 (2005): 43.

Page 174 *The American Cancer Society conducted a study*: H. S. Kahn, L. M. Tatham, C. Rodriguez, E. E. Calle, M. J. Thun, and C. W. Heath Jr., "Stable Behaviors Associated with Adults' 10-Year Change in Body Mass Index and Likelihood of Gain at the Waist," *American Journal of Public Health* 87, no. 5 (1997): 750.

Page 175 *The U.S. government's National Health and Nutrition Examination Survey*: Y. Papanikolaou and V. L. Fulgoni, "Bean Consumption Is Associated with Greater Nutrient

Intake, Reduced Systolic Blood Pressure, Lower Body Weight and a Smaller Waist Circumference in Adults: Results from the National Health and Nutrition Examination Survey, 1999–2002," *Journal of the American College of Nutrition* 27, no. 5 (2008): 573.

Page 176 *As my dear friend Dr. Janice Stanger*: J. Stanger, *The Perfect Formula Diet* (La Jolla, CA: Perfect Planet Solutions, 2009), p. 34.

Page 178 *Numerous studies, including the Harvard Nurses' Health Study*: D. Feskanich, W. C. Willet, M. J. Stampfer, and G. A. Colditz, "Milk, Dietary Calcium, and Bone Fractures in Women: A 12-Year Prospective Study," *American Journal of Public Health* 87 (1997): 996.

Page 179 *Researchers at Yale University found*: B. Abelow, "Cross-Cultural Association between Dietary Animal Protein and Hip Fracture: A Hypothesis," *Calcified Tissue International* 50 (1992): 15.

Page 179 *According to a study by Daniel Cramer, MD*: D. W. Cramer, B. L. Harlow, and W. C. Willet, "Galactose Consumption and Metabolism in Relation to the Risk of Ovarian Cancer," *Lancet* 2 (1989): 67.

Page 179 *Lactose intolerance affects approximately*: P. Bertron, N. D. Barnard, and M. Mills, "Racial Bias in Federal Nutrition Policy, Part I: The Public Health Implications of Variations in Lactase Persistence," *Journal of the National Medical Association* 91 (1999): 152.

Page 180 *In 1991, the World Health Organization*: World Health Organization, *Diet, Nutrition and the Prevention of Chronic Diseases*, WHO Technical Report Series 797 (Geneva: World Health Organization, 1991) and 916 (Geneva: World Health Organization, 2003).

Page 180 *In 1995, the Physicians Committee for Responsible Medicine*: Physicians Committee for Responsible Medicine, *Recommended Revisions for Dietary Guidelines for Americans* (Washington, DC: Physicians Committee for Responsible Medicine, January 31, 1995).

Page 180 *The following year, the Dietary Guidelines for Americans*: U.S. Department of Agriculture, Agricultural Research Service, Dietary Guidelines Advisory Committee, *Report of the Dietary Guidelines Advisory Committee on the Dietary Guidelines for Americans, 1995, to the Secretary of Health and Human Services and the Secretary of Agriculture* (Washington, DC: USDA, 1995), p. 22.

Page 180 *In 1997, the American Institute for Cancer Research*: World Cancer Research Fund and American Institute for Cancer Research, *Food, Nutrition, and the Prevention of Cancer: A Global Perspective* (Washington, DC: American Institute for Cancer Research, 1997).

Page 180 *And finally, in 2003, the American Dietetic Association*: A. R. Mangels et al., "Position of the American Dietetic Association and Dietitians of Canada: Vegetarian Diets," *Journal of the American Dietetic Association* 103, no. 6 (2003): 748.

Page 185 *A study of more than eighty-three thousand women*: "Nuts May Help Prevent Diabetes, Study of 83,000 Women Shows," *New York Times*, November 27, 2002.

Page 186 *An excellent book for addressing these conditions*: N. Barnard, *Dr. Neal Barnard's Program for Reversing Diabetes* (New York: Rodale, 2007).

Chapter Ten: Principle #3

Page 198 *John R. Lee, MD, author*: J. Lee and V. Hopkins, *What Your Doctor May Not Tell You about Premenopause: Balance Your Hormones and Your Life from Thirty to Fifty* (New York: Warner Books, 1999).

Page 210 *The allergist Theron Randolph, MD*: T. Randolph and R. Moss, *An Alternative Approach to Allergies* (New York: Bantam, 1980).

Page 210 *William H. Philpott, MD, and Dwight K. Kalita, PhD*: W. H. Philpott and D. K. Kalita, *Brain Allergies: The Psychonutrient Connection* (New Canaan, CT: Keats, 1987).

Page 215 *The most common rotation diet*: Herbert J. Rinkel, "Food Allergy IV: The Function and Clinical Application of the Rotary Diversified Diet," *Journal of Pediatrics* 32, no. 3 (1948): 266.

Chapter Eleven: Principle #4

Page 224 *The American College of Sports Medicine updated its physical activity guidelines*: C. E. Garber, B. Blissmer, M. Deschenes et al., "Quantity and Quality of Exercise for Developing and Maintaining Cardiorespiratory, Musculoskeletal, and Neuromotor Fitness in Apparently Healthy Adults: Guidance for Prescribing Exercise," *Medicine and Science in Sports and Exercise* 43, no. 7 (July 2011): 1334–59.

Page 225 *Adults should get at least 150 minutes*: American College of Sports Medicine news release, "ACSM Issues New Recommendations on Quantity and Quality of Exercise," August 1, 2011, www.acsm.org/about-acsm/media-room/news-releases/2011/08/01/acsm-issues-new-recommendations-on-quantity-and-quality-of-exercise.

Chapter Twelve: Principle #5

Page 236 *A 2006 study at Case Western Reserve University*: S. R. Patel, A. Malhotra, D. P. White et al., "Association between Reduced Sleep and Weight Gain in Women," *American Journal of Epidemiology* 164, no. 10 (2006): 952.

Page 237 *Lack of sleep leads to a rise in ghrelin*: K. Spiegel, E. Tasali, E. Van Cauter et al., "Brief Communication: Sleep Curtailment in Healthy Young Men Is Associated with Decreased Leptin Levels, Elevated Ghrelin Levels and Increased Hunger and Appetite," *Annals of Internal Medicine* 141 (2004): 848.

Page 239 *While individual needs may vary*: M. H. Bonnet and D. L. Arand, *How Much Sleep Do Adults Need?* (Arlington, VA: National Sleep Foundation, n.d.), www.sleepfoundation.org/article/white-papers/how-much-sleep-do-adults-need.

Chapter Thirteen: When Overeating Is Driven by Spiritual Hunger

Page 244 *Thomas Moore, an inspiring theologian*: T. Moore, *Care of the Soul* (New York: HarperCollins, 1992), pp. xii, 232, 5, xvi.

Chapter Fourteen: Practice #1

Page 252 *Eknath Easwaran, author*: E. Easwaran, *Meditation: Commonsense Directions for an Uncommon Life* (Petaluma, CA: Nilgiri Press, 1978), pp. 118.

Page 253 *One of my favorite inspirational passages*: For the origin of the Peace Prayer of St. Francis, see www.franciscan-archive.org/franciscana/peace.html.

Page 254 *Easwaran explains*: Easwaran, *Meditation*, p. 59.

Chapter Fifteen: Practice #2

Page 264 *Eckhart Tolle, spiritual teacher and author*: E. Tolle, *A New Earth: Awakening to Your Life's Purpose* (New York: Penguin, 2005), p. 43.

Page 266 *Shakti Gawain, author*: S. Gawain, *Creative Visualization* (New York: Bantam, 1978), p. 43.

Chapter Seventeen: Practice #4

Page 286 *John Cacioppo, a neuroscientist at the University of Chicago*: J. Cacioppo and W. Patrick, *Loneliness: Human Nature and the Need for Social Connection* (New York: W. W. Norton, 2008).

Bibliography

Aardal-Erikkson, E., B. E. Karlberg, and A. C. Holm. "Salivary Cortisol — an Alternative to Serum Cortisol Determinations in Dynamic Function Tests." *Clinical Chemistry and Laboratory Medicine* 36, no. 4 (April 1998): 215–22.

Acheson, K. "Carbohydrate Metabolism and de Novo Lipogenesis in Human Obesity." *American Journal of Clinical Nutrition* 45 (1987): 78.

———. "Glycogen Storage Capacity and de Novo Lipogenesis during Massive Carbohydrate Overfeeding in Man." *American Journal of Clinical Nutrition* 48 (1988): 240.

Appleton, N. *Lick the Sugar Habit*. Garden City, NY: Avery, 1997.

Arem, R. *The Thyroid Solution: A Revolutionary Mind-Body Program for Regaining Your Emotional and Physical Health*. New York: Random House, 2007.

Barnard, N. *Dr. Neal Barnard's Program for Reversing Diabetes*. New York: Rodale, 2007.

Berg, F. M. *The Health Risks of Weight Loss*. Hettinger, ND: Healthy Living Institute, 1993.

Blackburn, G. L., et al. "Weight Cycling: The Experience of Human Dieters." *American Journal of Clinical Nutrition* 49 (1989): 1105.

Braly, J., and P. Holford. *Hidden Food Allergies: The Essential Guide to Uncovering Hidden Food Allergies and Achieving Permanent Relief*. London: Piatkus Books, 2005.

Braverman, E. *The Edge Effect*. New York: Sterling, 2005.

Braverman, E., and C. Pfeiffer. *The Healing Nutrients Within*. New Canaan, CT: Keats, 1997.

Cass, H., and P. Holford. *Natural Highs*. New York: Penguin, 2002.

Cousens, G. *Depression Free for Life*. New York: HarperCollins, 2001.

Craig, G. *EFT for Weight Loss*. Fulton, CA: Energy Psychology Press, 2010.

De Stefani, E., A. Ronco, M. Mendilaharsu, et al. "Meat Intake, Heterocyclic Amines, and Risk of Breast Cancer: A Case-Control Study in Uruguay." *Cancer Epidemiology, Biomarkers and Prevention* 6 (1997): 573–81.

Duncan, K. "The Effects of High and Low Energy Density Diets on Satiety, Energy Intake, and Eating Time of Obese and Nonobese Subjects. *American Journal of Clinical Nutrition* 37 (1983): 763.

Ellis, A. *A New Guide to Rational Living*. North Hollywood, CA: Wilshire Books, 1975.

"Ethics Opinion: Weight Loss Products and Medications." *Journal of the American Dietetic Association* 108 (2008): 2109–13.

Fuhrman, J. *Eat to Live*. Boston: Little, Brown, 2003.

Gaesser, G. A. *Big Fat Lies: The Truth about Your Weight and Your Health*. New York: Ballantine Books, 1998.

Giovannuci, E., and B. Goldin. "The Role of Fat, Fatty Acids, and Total Energy Intake in the Etiology of Human Colon Cancer." *American Journal of Clinical Nutrition* 66, no. 6 (1997): 1564–71S.

Horwath, N. C., E. Saltzman, and S. B. Roberts. "Dietary Fiber and Weight Regulation." *Nutrition Reviews* 59 (2001): 129–39.

Johnson, P. M., and P. J. Kenny. "Dopamine D2 Receptors in Addiction-Like Reward Dysfunction and Compulsive Eating in Obese Rats." *Nature Neuroscience* 13 (2010): 635–41.

Kessler, D. A. *The End of Overeating*. New York: Rodale, 2009.

Knight, E. L., et al. "The Impact of Protein Intake on Renal Function Decline in Women with Normal Renal Function or Mild Renal Insufficiency." *Annals of Internal Medicine* 138 (2003): 460–67.

Kress, Diane. *The Metabolism Miracle*. Philadelphia: Da Capo Press, 2009.

Lee, J., and V. Hopkins. *What Your Doctor May Not Tell You about Menopause: The Breakthrough Book on Natural Progesterone*. New York: Warner Books, 1996.

LeShan, L. *How to Meditate*. Boston: Little, Brown, 1974.

Lieberman, H. "The Effects of Dietary Neurotransmitter Precursors on Human Behavior." *American Journal of Clinical Nutrition* 42 (1985): 366.

Lisle, D. J., and A. Goldhamer. *The Pleasure Trap*. Summertown, TN: Healthy Living Publications, 2003.

Lissner, L., et al. "Variability of Body Weight and Health Outcomes in the Framingham Population." *New England Journal of Medicine* 324 (1991): 1839–44.

Mann T., and A. J. Tomiyama, et al. "Medicare's Search for Effective Obesity Treatments: Diets Are Not the Answer." *American Psychology* 62 (2007): 220–33.

McDougall, J. "Resisting the Broken Bone Businesses: Bone Mineral Density Tests and the Drugs That Follow." *McDougall Newsletter* 3, no. 10 (October 2004), www.neal hendrickson.com/McDougall/2004nl/041000.htm.

Miller, W. C. "How Effective Are Traditional Dietary and Exercise Interventions for Weight Loss?" *Medicine and Science in Sports Exercise* 31 (1999): 1129–34.

Moore, R. Y. "Circadian Rhythms: Basic Neurobiology and Clinical Applications." *Annual Review of Medicine* 48 (1997): 253–66.

Murray, M. *Premenstrual Syndrome*. Rocklin, CA: Prima, 1997.

National Heart, Lung, and Blood Institute. *Restless Legs Syndrome: Detection and Management in Primary Care*. NIH Pub. No. 00-3788. Bethesda, MD: NHLBI, 2000.

————. *Sleep Apnea: Is Your Patient at Risk?* NIH Pub. No. 99-3803. Reprint. 1995; Bethesda, MD: NHLBI, 1999.

Papanikolaou, Y., et al. "Bean Consumption by Adults Is Associated with a More Nutrient Dense Diet and a Reduced Risk of Obesity." Presented at the Experimental Biology Conference, April 1–5, 2006, San Francisco.

Potter, J. D. "Nutrition and Colorectal Cancer." *Cancer Causes Control* 7, no. 1 (1996): 127–46.

Purba, M., and M. Grundmann-Killmann. "Low Molecular Weight Antioxidants and Their Role in Skin Aging." *Clinical and Experimental Dermatology* 26 (2001): 578–82.

Rapp, D. *Is This Your Child? Discovering and Treating Unrecognized Allergies in Children and Adults*. New York: William Morrow, 1992.

Rivera, R., and F. Deutsch. *Your Hidden Food Allergies Are Making You Fat*. Rocklin, CA: Prima, 1998.

Ross, J. *The Diet Cure*. New York: Penguin, 1999.

————. *The Mood Cure*. New York: Penguin, 2002.

Ryde, D., and T. Wardle. *Your Health in Your Hands*, 2007, Vegetarian and Vegan Foundation, www.vegetarian.org.uk/guides/yourhealth.html.

Saunders, K. *The Vegan Diet*. New York: Lantern Books, 2003.

Schwarzbein, D. *The Schwarzbein Principle: The Program*. Deerfield Beach, FL: Health Communications, 2004.

Shames, R., and K. Shames. *Feeling Fat, Fuzzy, or Frazzled? A Three-Step Program to Restore Thyroid, Adrenal, and Reproductive Balance*. London: Penguin, 2005.

Shapiro, F. *EMDR: Eye Movement Desensitization and Reprocessing: Basic Principles, Protocols, and Procedures*. New York: Guilford Press, 2001.

Shell, E. R. *The Hungry Gene*. New York: Atlantic Monthly Press, 2002.

Slagle, P. *The Way Up from Down*. New York: St. Martin's Press, 1994.

Stanger, J. *The Perfect Formula Diet*. La Jolla, CA: Perfect Planet Solutions, 2009.

Titchenal, C. A., J. C. Dobbs, and R. K. Hetzler. "Macronutrient Composition of the Zone Diet Based on Computer Analysis." *Medicine and Science in Sports and Exercise* 29, no. 5 (1997): S126.

Tribole, E., and E. Resch. *Intuitive Eating*. New York: St. Martin's Press, 2003.

Vliet, E. *Screaming to Be Heard: Hormonal Connections Women Suspect and Doctors Ignore*. New York: Evans, 1995.

Waterhouse, D. *Outsmarting the Midlife Fat Cell*. New York: Hyperion Books, 1998.

Weil, A. *Natural Health, Natural Medicine*. Boston: Houghton Mifflin, 1998.

Westman, E. C., et al. "Effect of a 6-Month Adherence to a Very Low Carbohydrate Diet Program." *American Journal of Medicine* 113 (2002): 30–36.

Wilson, J. L. *Adrenal Fatigue: The 21st Century Stress Syndrome*. Petaluma, CA: Smart Publications, 2001.

Wurtman, J. "Carbohydrate Craving in Obese People: Suppression by Treatments Affecting Serotoninergic Transmission." *International Journal of Eating Disorders* 1, no. (1981): 2.

Index

T

About the Author

Julie M. Simon, MA, MBA, LMFT, is a licensed psychotherapist and life coach with more than twenty years of experience helping overeaters stop dieting, heal their relationships with themselves and their bodies, lose excess weight, and keep it off. A lifelong fitness enthusiast, she is also a certified personal trainer with over twenty-five years of experience designing exercise and nutrition programs for various populations. Julie is also the founder and director of the Los Angeles–based Twelve-Week Emotional Eating Recovery Program, which offers an alternative to dieting by addressing the mind, body, and spirit imbalances underlying overeating. Her professional experience with and personal journey through childhood trauma, weight challenges, and body, brain, and spiritual imbalances led to the creation of the twelve-week program, which she has been running for twenty years. She is also the creator of the Women Who Eat for Emotional Comfort support groups.

For over two decades, Julie has presented seminars and workshops on overcoming overeating, and on associated mental health topics, to both lay and professional audiences, for the UCLA Staff and Faculty Counseling Center, the Santa Monica College Continuing Education and Community Services, the Learning Annex, the Los Angeles Dietetic Association, the YMCA, and Whole Foods markets, among others.

Julie formerly served for many years on the board of the Los Angeles Chapter of the California Association of Marriage and Family Therapists in different capacities. She lives and practices in Los Angeles.

For more information and inspiration,
visit Julie's website at www.overeatingrecovery.com.